Cosmetics
FROM THE
Kitchen

MARCIA DONNAN

HOLT, RINEHART AND WINSTON
New York   Chicago   San Francisco

Published simultaneously in Canada by HOLT, RINEHART
AND WINSTON OF CANADA, LIMITED.

ISBN: 0-03-091893-6

Library of Congress Catalog Card Number: 72-78125

Published, October, 1972
Second Printing, March, 1973

Designer: Betty Binns

PRINTED IN THE UNITED STATES OF AMERICA

To Jack, my favorite chemist;

to Alan and Krissy,
my favorite kitchen assistants;

to my mother,
my favorite proofreader;

and to Dr. Gertrude Witherspoon Moore,
who first interested us in cosmetic chemistry.

Contents

Preface   *xiii*

1 **From the Nile to Hollywood**   *1*

2 **Why Cosmetics?**   *10*

3 **Making Your Own Cosmetics**   *14*

4 **Cosmetic Safety**   *20*

5 **Basic Instructions for Formulating Cosmetics in the Kitchen**   *25*

6 **Perfumes, Colors, and Preservatives**   *33*

7 **Caring for the Skin**   *40*

CREAMS 48
Basic Cold Cream No. 1   Basic Cold Cream No. 2   Basic Cold Cream No. 3   Theatrical Cold Cream   All-Purpose Cream   Cleansing Cream No. 1   Cleansing Cream No. 2   Liquid Cleansing Cream   Cleansing Lotion   Cleansing Milk   Simple Vanishing Cream   Dry-Skin Vanishing Cream   Avocado Moisturizer Lubricating Cream

SKIN LOTIONS 59
Astringent Lotion   Skin Freshener

MASKS 60
Kaolin Mask   Gelatin Mask

HAND CREAMS AND LOTIONS   62
*Simple Hand Cream (Oily)   Glycerin and
Rose Water   Avocado Cream   Deluxe Hand
Cream*

POWDERS   65
Baby Powder   Talcum Powders

TANNING PREPARATIONS   67
Sun Tan Oil   Sun Tan Cream

8   **Hormones and Vitamins**   *69*

9   **Preparations to Beautify**   *76*

FACE MAKEUP   87
*Foundation Cream   Pigmented Foundation
Cream   Cream Makeup   Liquid Makeup
Face Powders   Blush Rouge   Lipstick*

EYE MAKEUP   96
*Cream Eye Shadow   Powder Eye Shadow
Cake Mascara No. 1   Cake Mascara No. 2
Mascara Crayon   Eye Makeup Remover*

NAIL PREPARATIONS   102
Nail Buffing Paste   Nail Polish Remover

FRAGRANCES   104
*Homemade Perfumes   Cream Cologne
"Pure Joy"*

10   **Preparations for Grooming**   *107*

HAIR PREPARATIONS   114
*Liquid Shampoo   Cream Shampoo   Simple
Oil Shampoo   Soap Shampoo   Hot Oil
Conditioner   Hair-Set Preparation*

MOUTH PREPARATIONS   120
Toothpaste   Tooth Powder   Mouthwash

DEODORANTS AND ANTI-PERSPIRANTS   122
*Anti-perspirant Cream   Liquid Anti-
perspirant*

BATH PREPARATIONS 123
*Foam Bath   Bath Oil   Bath Salts   Body
Oil*

11   There's a Man in the Kitchen *127*

HAIR PREPARATIONS 133
Hair Cream   Clear Hairdressing

SHAVING PREPARATIONS 134
*Brushless Shaving Cream No. 1   Brushless
Shaving Cream No. 2   Electric Pre-shave
Lotion   After-shave Stick   After-shave Lotion*

HAND PREPARATIONS 138
*Extra-rich Hand Lubricant   Hand Cleaner
No. 1   Hand Cleaner No. 2*

CREAMS 141
*Protective Sun Cream   Mentholated Cream
for Massage*

DEODORANTS 142
Deodorant Stick   Deodorant Foot Powder

PERFUME 143
Men's Cologne

Appendix A: Definitions and Sources of Supply 147
Appendix B: Suppliers 162
Index 167

Preface

Not long ago an executive of a cosmetics manufacturing firm was asked for help in finding a rather unusual cosmetic ingredient. In answer to his question about why in the world anyone would want to buy *that* particular material, he was told that the author needed it for a cosmetic she was making in her kitchen.

"Anyone can make most of them in a kitchen," he admitted. "Someday women are going to realize this."

Some of them already do—but most do not. Some have taken courses in the chemistry of cosmetics, but found that formulas written in the metric system and the need for sophisticated equipment meant that their new-found knowledge was of little use outside the college laboratory.

We are speaking of honest-to-goodness cosmetic preparations, not those made at home from a variety of fresh fruits and vegetables. Researching the works of some of the most prestigious chemists in the field leads us to wonder about the benefit of these foods used as cosmetics, although their concentrated oils and juices are sometimes beneficial in certain preparations. It occurs to us that piling sliced bananas, orange pulp, and grapefruit on the skin might make a woman delicious looking for the moment, but there is some question about long-range benefits. It might be fun to look like a fruit salad, but, on the other hand, an unsuspected allergy might make the next course hives.

And so the cosmetics included here are the traditional preparations used to cleanse, beautify, and groom the body—oils and creams that soothe, pamper, and delay the signs of aging. There are excellent preparations to beautify: lipstick, powder, makeup, and eye preparations. They are made of the finest ingredients and truly are bargains for those who wish to make them at home. Some date back many years (almost to antiquity), others are as modern as today, and all, without exception, offer the opportunity for a totally individualistic approach to beauty.

Formulas are in "kitchenese," the familiar language of the kitchen, and use the tools of that same happy place: measuring cups and spoons, spatulas, a cheese grater, and pots and pans. Techniques of manufacture are explained in step-by-step directions with each formula and in Chapter 5, "Basic Instructions for Formulating Cosmetics in the Kitchen."

Savings involved in home manufacture of cosmetics are substantial. For fun, we calculated the cost of making a fine lubricating cream—20¢. One would expect to pay at least $4 for a preparation of similar quality on the market. Most ingredients are inexpensive and many are as near as the corner drugstore, grocery store, or health food store.

How do you know exactly what to buy and where to buy it? Check the appendices in the back of this book for information on ingredients and sources of supply. Included are names and addresses of major suppliers of cosmetic ingredients and laboratory equipment.

To the person who enjoys creating, and who is truly an individual, the author issues an invitation to begin making cosmetics. Rich creams and other preparations make lovely gifts, and the person who first showers family and friends with cosmetics from the kitchen will gain a new status—something between gourmet cook and artist.

What's cooking?

Cosmetics!

MARCIA DONNAN

Hill City, South Dakota
March 1972

Cosmetics
FROM THE
Kitchen

1

From the Nile to Hollywood

A HISTORY OF COSMETICS

Cleopatra, back in 50 B.C., prepared herself for a typical day of political intrigue by painting a generous amount of black *kohl* above her eyes, stroking green *kohl* below them, thickening her dark lashes and brows with more of the black substance made from antimony, and by being rubbed with fragrant, soothing oils. If the legendary queen of the Egyptians was not beautiful when she completed her preparations (and there are those writers of the past who insist she was not), she was at least one of the most glamorous women of any era.

History, since its beginnings, tells us that women of all levels of social and economic status have sought the means of becoming beautiful. If certain oils and cosmetics were rare and expensive, there were others that were not, and even the poorest peasant woman found a way to protect and smooth her skin and to improve her appearance.

Attitudes about beauty reflected feelings about self and society, and in various countries during various periods of history, women (and sometimes men) painted and powdered and padded one year and became very Puritan about it all the next. But throughout, and even during the most austere times, oils and ointments have been used to care for the skin, and certain other preparations were concocted to aid, if ever so subtly, in the search for beauty.

While modern science tackles with ease such seemingly incredible chores as dating ancient rocks and accurately plotting the course of the earth's voyage through history, it cannot tell us much about the early stages of the manufacture of cosmetics and perfumes. Chemical analysis of cosmetics presents great difficulties, even with products manufactured today. To this dismal outlook for accurate analysis, add the factor of time—and the chemist is lost before he begins. Over the years, chemical action has altered the constitution of ancient preparations, effectively guarding their secrets from modern-day researchers.

We know more about why and how cosmetics were used by ancient peoples than we know about the cosmetics themselves. Many of the terms used by the ancients to make their cosmetics remain unidentified, and chemical analyses of unguents and other cosmetics unearthed in tombs yield few clues to their original formulations. Still, there is some knowledge of the basic materials used, gained through writings by later Greek and Roman authors.

It is interesting to learn about some of the basics used in early cosmetics, even if we don't know exactly how they were used or in what proportions. Many of them are quite familiar, and some are used today, making ancient glamour something not *entirely* mysterious.

Olive oil and castor oil were typically used by the poorer people, as well as ben oil, radish oil, colocynth oil, and sesame oil. There was nothing very rare about these oils and most everyone had access to them. Perfumes and flavors included those of bitter almond, aniseed, calamus, cassia, cedar, cinnamon, citron, ginger, heliotrope, mimosa, peppermint, rose, rosemary, rushes, sandalwood, and gingergrass.

If it seems distasteful that ox, sheep, and goose fats were used in early cosmetics, consider that lanolin, an extremely valuable constituent of modern cosmetics, is extracted from wool. And if the jars, tubes, and bottles of cosmetics we buy all carried lists of ingredients (such as those found on sausages), we might find a number of items that would disturb us even more than ox and goose fats.

What about fragrances?

Henna flowers, iris roots, honey, wine, and other good things no longer used in the art of perfumery were onetime favorites of early perfumers. The Near Eastern perfumers were unable to make use of musk, ambergris, and civet—all inaccessible in that part of the world.

Physical evidence of the existence and use of ancient cosmetics comes mainly from archeological finds of toilet

articles and unguents. When Howard Carter opened the
tomb of Tutankhamen, who ruled about 1350 B.C., he
found more than royal remains. Eyewitnesses to the
historic event are reported to have seen—and smelled—
unguent vases containing quantities of aromatics that
were still fragrant.

There were even earlier cosmetic finds, with some
dated as far back as 3500 B.C.

Although the possibility that cosmetic art began in
China is a very real one, solid evidence of its beginning
is found in Egypt. The fact that the ancient Egyptians
placed great value on cosmetics, including them in their
burial paraphernalia, makes it possible for us to learn
something about the ancient art.

It was not unheard of for the Egyptian man on the
street to insist upon a fair ration of cosmetics. During
the reign of King Rameses III, workers in the Theban
necropolis went out on strike because, they said, they
lacked sufficient ointment. No one, it seemed, should
have to work under such awful conditions. There was no
doubt that the ancient Egyptians accepted as fact the
necessity of using ointments and aromatic oils for all
classes of people.

In ancient Israel, feelings about cosmetics appear to
have been inconsistent. One reads that "ointment and
perfume rejoice the heart" (Prov. XXVII. 9), but one
also reads how the prophet curses the son of the sor-
ceress: "Thou wentest to the King with ointment, and
didst increase thy perfumes . . . and didst debase thy-
self even unto hell" (Isa. LVII. 9).

Cosmetics and perfumes were frequently and freely

used by the Assyrians, Babylonians, Sumerians, and Syrians. These peoples seem to have been less enthusiastic about bathing than were the Egyptians, however, for bathtubs were used only by the rich. As for the Mesopotamians, they were said to have washed the body only on very special occasions. Use of cosmetics by some peoples had little to do with thoughts about keeping clean.

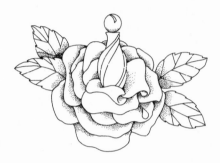

The history of cosmetics is inextricably involved with that of religion, medicine, and magic. While ancient peoples—especially those living in hot, dry climates— soon learned the value of protective oils, use of oils was not solely cosmetic. During the period of King Thutmose IV, special unguents had great religious significance and were made only by the priests, with formulas that were carefully guarded secrets. One Egyptian papyrus leaves no doubt that priests had sole distribution rights for these precious cosmetics.

In the New Testament, a most familiar passage tells how unguents were carried to the tomb of Christ to anoint his dead body. This is only one of many biblical references to anointment, a means of consecrating through application of oils.

There is abundant historical evidence of magical elements in the use of early cosmetics. The warrior who had his body rubbed with oil before going into battle was seeking supernatural support for the struggle ahead, not improving his appearance for the gang on the other side of the river.

Gradually, religious and magical meanings gave way to practical ones, and cosmetics began to be used more for beautifying than for anything else.

From the beginning, however, we can be certain that there were those clever females who knew the value of soft skin and sweet-smelling bodies. They probably understood more about the real magic of cosmetics than the priests.

One can well believe that Egyptian women who experimented with cosmetics did so to enhance their beauty. During Cleopatra's time crude paints were used with great skill by Egyptian women, especially for the eyes. But they also painted lips and cheeks, usually with red ocher. A red pigment from henna was applied to hair and nails. The fashionable ladies of Mesopotamia also used red ocher, asafetida, and henna, but the Sumerian women preferred yellow for their cheeks.

Eye disease was a problem among the Egyptians, and so it followed that eye makeup originally had properties that would allow it to serve a medicinal purpose. But, as paint became more popular for its cosmetic value, the nature of the preparation changed—a typical evolution for certain cosmetics.

History assures us that the hand that rocked the Cradle of Civilization was softened with oils and scented with perfumes. In other parts of the world and at other times, societies soon "discovered" the use of cosmetics.

Busy with other matters, the Romans paid little notice to cosmetics until they moved into the area of southern Italy occupied by the Greeks. Then it was a good thing to be shared, and by the time of Nero, painting and powdering was definitely the thing to do. White lead and chalk whitened skin, Egyptian *kohl* darkened eyelids and lashes, fucus (rouge) was used on lips and cheeks, psilotrum was used as a depilatory, barley flour, and butter were applied to discourage blemishes, and the prettiest Romans around were those whose teeth were polished with pumice stone.

The crusaders brought secrets of the Near Eastern harem back to Britain and their womenfolk were delighted with the fragrant cosmetics. Sweet coffers held the cosmetics owned by the ladies of the realm and were considered a necessary part of the furnishings of the bedroom. Lovely complexions during the time of Elizabeth I were thought to come from a brisk rubdown with wine following a steaming bath. For those less fortunate, milk had to suffice.

That British women indulged in cosmetics to a degree some thought immoral is evidenced in the bill introduced in Parliament in 1770:

That all women, whatever age, rank, profession or degree, whether virgins, maids, or widows, that shall, from and after such Act, impose upon, seduce, and betray into matrimony, any of his Majesty's subjects, by the scents, paints, cosmetic washes, artificial teeth, false hair, Spanish wool, iron stays, hoops, high-heeled shoes, bolstered hips, shall incur the penalty of the law in force against witchcraft and like misdemeanors and that the marriage, upon confliction, shall stand null and void.

It was hardly a climate for thoughts of women's liberation.

At the time the young colony of Pennsylvania adopted the same law, the use of cosmetics was frowned upon in most American colonies. The fact is that the history of using cosmetics in this country parallels closely that of Europe. During colonial times such use varied in different parts of the country, depending upon the social climate in a particular area. In Puritan New England, cosmetics were banned on moral grounds; in the southern colonies of French origin, cosmetics were used freely.

It is a matter of social history that not until after World War I were cosmetics considered acceptable by most well-bred Americans. The image of the "painted lady" persists even today among some of the more conservative, rural communities and within certain religious groups.

In Italy, France, and Spain, cosmetics also went through on-again, off-again popularity, mainly due to the whims of rulers reigning at the time. France's Louis XIII approved and cosmetics were popular; Louis XIV disapproved and they were unpopular.

From ancient times to modern, through religious, magical, medicinal, and social influences, women—and men—have artificially changed their appearances for one reason or another. The reason now is the search for beauty, and women are learning that it is possible to effect a real change not only in looks but in the health of skin, hair, nails, and teeth through wise use of cosmetics. From Cleopatra's eyes to Elizabeth's wine rub to Clara Bow's rouge circles to Twiggy's lashes, the name of the game (and the prize) has been beauty.

Not all women are willing to go to the lengths revealed by Princess Luciana Pignatelli, who wrote of not only extensive beauty preparations and techniques but of undergoing artificial implantation for the sake of being beautiful. But most women realize they can be truly lovelier to others and to themselves through wise use of cosmetics.

Scientific research makes it possible to live longer. There is no reason why it shouldn't make us look better while we are doing it.

2

Why Cosmetics?

Was the red-haired mummy of Hentawi (18th Dynasty) something of a vamp? Possibly, for at some period during her life she had decided to be a redhead even though that was not nature's plan. It is more likely, however, that she was an ordinary woman who realized the benefits of helping nature along through the use of cosmetics.

As the lifespan increases, so does the need to keep the skin and hair healthy, lovely to look at, and as youthful as possible. Why? Not because of vanity, but because a person feels better when she (or he) looks better.

Proper diet and exercise, good health habits, and an abundance of other factors contribute to staying—and looking—younger longer. A major factor is keeping the external body healthy and attractive through using quality preparations that cleanse, lubricate, and beautify.

The why of cosmetics is involved with the why of enjoying the finer possibilities of life. Putting a best face forward makes for a better day and greater accomplishment.

Early in World War II, British manufacture of cosmetics was curtailed to 25 percent of normal production. Women working in factories drooped through their days, and morale steadily declined. When cosmetic stations were set up in the factories, morale soared. A U.S. report,* citing the phenomenon, notes, "the effect was so striking that the restricting order for the nation as a whole was relaxed to 50 percent of the peacetime level" of cosmetics manufacture.

Looking your best tells others something of how you feel about your own worth. The carefully wrapped lady of Hentawi sent a message over 3000 years old when archaeologists found evidence of red hair dye, a message that said she cared about how she looked.

Cosmetics protect as well as beautify. A good moisturizing lipstick prevents chapped lips; lubricating creams with lanolin bathe the skin with the best substitute for natural oils, effectively replacing those lost through drying and aging processes; vanishing creams and makeup protect the skin from the weather. Hair preparations restore natural oils and body to dry hair; buffing with an old-fashioned nail cream can make nails stronger and keep them healthy and lovely. There are bountiful rewards that come from *good* cosmetics properly used.

* Report of the Office of Civilian Supply to the U.S. Director of Economic Stabilization (1943).

In the good old days, someone is certain to say, "a natural bristle hair brush and homemade soap were enough." In those same good old days in America, most women were haggard by the age of twenty-five and dead by the age of thirty-five. There is no reason to reflect on the romance of a period when baths were a once-a-month luxury and skin was dry and leathery. Besides, half the work of cosmetics is in cleansing and protecting, and few can argue the value of that.

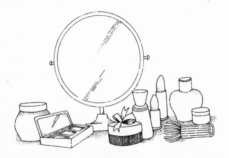

Why cosmetics? Why not?

One "why not" offered now and again is the cost of preparations made from inexpensive ingredients, packaged in handsome, gilt-trimmed containers, and sold for the price of a week's food budget. It is a good point to raise, and one that women should raise more frequently than they do. There is not all that much in a name, and if a rich, homemade lubricating cream can do the job, there is certainly no need for an exotic formulation that won't do any more.

When should a girl begin to use cosmetics? The 13-year-old who has a penchant for deep purple eye shadow, false eyelashes, and blood-red lips should be treated to a

trip to a cosmetic salon to find out what cosmetics are all about. During those early teen years, it is well to start a lifetime habit of care of the skin, hair, and nails and to begin some subtle experimentation with the basics of cosmetics. The face a youngster shows to the rest of her world tells more about her than anything she can say, and clean, well-cared-for skin, a bright and white smile, and shiny clean hair say a lot more for her than the purple eyes—something anyone but her mother can explain to her.

The thing to remember, at any age, is that improper use of cosmetics can do as much damage as neglect. Hair that is treated, dyed, permanently waved, and tortured over and over again is going to fall out (or break off) faster than hair that is totally neglected. Makeup layered on an unclean skin day after day can result in a complexion that looks as if it belongs to the Witch of the North Woods. Eye irritation can come from eye makeup blobbed indiscriminately here and there about the eyes, and certain tanning preparations can leave a girl looking like a leopard.

But cosmetics, properly used, can give a new lease on life. They can disguise minor disfigurations and make a plain Jane someone very special. It takes very little time, and sometimes the advice of a professional, to learn the ins and outs of cosmetic care. It is worth it, however, in terms of added years of looking younger and feeling better.

For many a woman, the fountain of youth springs from her own cosmetics cabinet.

3

Making Your Own Cosmetics

It is a do-it-yourself world peopled by individuals who are no longer going to buy a new convertible because the Joneses just bought one. The new attitude about living and buying is what the consumer revolution is all about, according to consumer specialists studying this phenomenon now affecting the nation's purchasers of goods and services.

Americans are finding their own life-styles and being bold about it. They are impatient with and not taken in by elaborate advertising schemes designed to mold them into a nation of be-alikes. They are more individualistic in their ideas and their actions than any of their ancestors have been.

It's a healthy kind of revolution, and one that brings

great rewards to those who are a part of it. Home sewing is at its peak during this period of American fashion history. The man next door is building his own fireplace and his wife is polishing stones for her own jewelry.

And so it follows that women, who spend a small fortune on creams and makeup during their lifetimes, and men, who are great do-it-yourselfers, might want to make their own beautifying and grooming preparations. With many ingredients available at the local drugstore, and equipment as simple as a measuring cup and an egg beater, there is no reason why they shouldn't be able to whip up a batch of lanolin-rich lubricating cream that is at least as good as the one they have been buying at many times the price of the homemade product.

The most exciting thing about making cosmetics is that it is fun. Watching an emulsion take place is far more thrilling than beating up a creamy cake frosting. "Cooking" cosmetics in the kitchen is as rewarding, and usually far less tiring, than putting together a gourmet meal.

A woman who makes her own cosmetics can be totally individualistic about her appearance. Her creams can be perfect for her skin, her makeup colors uniquely her own. The man in her life will enjoy every bit as much being individualistic about the grooming products he uses, including a favorite he-man scent (or not so he-man, if he chooses). Further, the do-it-yourself cosmeticologist knows exactly what ingredients go into each preparation, what they cost, and what their contribution is to the final product.

As for money saved, it will take a while to compute exact dollars and cents savings. This much is unquestioned—after the initial cost of buying some of the basic ingredients, you are in the business of creating your own cosmetics at an astonishingly low cost.

Another reward in making cosmetics in the kitchen comes from the very business of creating—the same kind of reward that comes to potters, artists, and those whose joy of living comes from within.

And speaking of joy, included in this volume is the formula for a perfume reported to be a "twin" to Jean Patou's famed and expensive ($65 an ounce) "Joy." You can make it for $3. This copycat formula is called "Pure Joy."

Cosmetic formulas change from time to time, either because a different ingredient improves the effectiveness, appearance, or stability of the preparation, or because a change provides the opportunity to advertise an exciting new cosmetic—a far less lofty reason.

Many of the formulas used in this book are several years old. These are the simpler formulas, ones easy to make which use ingredients readily available at the corner drugstore. The rest are more "modern" formulations, occasionally more complex or using ingredients you *may* have to special order.

In spite of the aura of mystery that still surrounds the formulation of cosmetics, there is very little that is mysterious about the whole thing. For example, researching the most prestigious half-dozen formularies used around the world will point to the fact that ideas about cold creams or vanishing creams or foundation makeups are very much the same. Variations in proportions and in the use of similar ingredients make the difference between one formulation and another. In selecting the formulas for this book we had to choose from hundreds that are similar, many of which we have used for years. Where we had three formulas for vanishing creams that were almost identical, we selected the one that had an outstanding feature, such as extra-fine texture. This is all part of the fun of making cosmetics—trying formulas and deciding which is most pleasing to you. From those given in this book you will want to choose a wardrobe of cosmetics tailor-made to suit your needs.

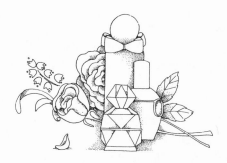

The proof of the cosmetic is in the using. Old or new, whatever is most effective must be the best formula.

Don't discard some of the way-back-when formulas until you have given them a try. Nothing can beat Grandmother's glycerine and rose water for the loveliest, smoothest hands in town. Soaking fingers for five minutes in a bowl of this heavenly stuff means no more hangnails and suddenly beautiful cuticles. Treating the hands to a frequent massage with this age-old cosmetic will do more for you than the most expensive and richest hand cream on the market.

Another leftover from the Stutz Bearcat crowd is

the practice of nail buffing with a nail paste. For many, it cures splitting, layering, and chipping nails, and promotes growth far better than a lifetime supply of gelatin. And it is a lot easier on the appetite.

The author has spent many hours making cosmetics in the kitchen—never for sale, but for personal use and for gifts. During college days she was a reader for a course in the chemistry of cosmetics, assisting the professor and working in the laboratory. Cleverly, she married the chemistry major who was the laboratory assistant for the course.

Rest assured it isn't necessary to have a husband who is a chemist if you want to make cosmetics in the kitchen. But if you want to *experiment* with cosmetics, then you had better check over the chemistry majors in the neighborhood.

In this book we have included the formulas we have used and enjoyed—formulas that are safe, effective, and that produce cosmetics as fine as any in the world. You can pay higher prices for cosmetics, but you won't find safer, higher quality preparations anywhere.

It is important to remember that in manufacturing your own cosmetics, ingredients must be properly measured and instructions carefully followed. If a formula calls for 4 ounces of material, it does not mean 4 ounces more or less. These are honest-to-goodness chemical formulas, not recipes for split pea soup (although we frequently refer to them as "recipes"), and the practice of "a pinch of this, a pinch of that" must be abandoned— unless, of course, the formula calls for a pinch, which some do. In a case where experimentation is permissible, the formula will say so—for example, "Increasing the ratio of beeswax to mineral oil and water will stiffen the cream. . . ."

In *all* cases, follow instructions. They are simple and sure-fire if they are adhered to by kitchen cosmeticologists.

4

Cosmetic Safety

When you manufacture cosmetics at home, for your own use or for gifts, are you breaking the law? Can a policeman invade your kitchen and snatch your cleansing cream?

He cannot.

While the manufacture and distribution of cosmetics are strictly regulated (thank goodness), it is only the products made and distributed *for sale* that are affected by legally established regulatory measures.

What about this business of manufacturing your own cosmetics—just how safe is it? How safe can you consider your products to be? As long as no one is going to be standing over your shoulder with a book of rules, how do you know that what you have made will be harmless to skin and health?

First of all, there is no assurance that *any* cosmetic, no matter how carefully prepared or by whom, is 100 percent safe for 100 percent of the people who will use it. Laws regulating commercial manufacture of cosmetics recognize this, for even if isolated complaints come in against certain products, those products may still be judged safe for *general* use and be retained on the market. So one must consider that the ultimate safety of cosmetics (either "store bought" or homemade) must be viewed from the aspect of *general* usage. Most all persons using the formulas in this book will find them not only fun to make but safe to use as well. Homemade products should not be considered any more hazardous than those purchased every day in the stores, for essentially, ingredients and formulation are the same.

An important consideration here lies in following directions and, especially, in purchasing the exact ingredients called for. Many ingredients will be labeled USP (United States Pharmacopeia) or NF (National Formulary) grades; others will not be so labeled. Ask your pharmacist's advice, and heed it, when it comes to buying ingredients. *In general* do not use "technical" grade, for this denotes ingredients not sufficiently pure for drug use. But do ask the pharmacist if you have questions about ingredients. Tell him what you are doing—making cosmetics at home—and if he is anything like the druggists we've worked with through the years, he will be as interested in helping you secure the right ingredients as you are in buying them.

The chapter "Perfumes, Colors, and Preservatives" discusses in detail the safety of dyes. Here again, following directions and buying specified ingredients assures you that your finished products should be safe to use.

Some of the formulas in this book use ingredients from way-back-when. Mineral oil, borax, beeswax, and the like were the basics for cosmetics when Grandma was trying to entice Grandpa to the altar. Buying cosmetic grades of the old standbys is always a safe way to go; however, newer products which may provide improved stability, texture, or effectiveness should not be considered unsafe because they have not been around for centuries. New ingredients undergo intensive and extensive testing by the manufacturers long before they are put on the market.

If a kitchen cosmeticologist decides to try writing her own formulas and ends up with something resembling an Old English pox, we can only sigh and offer our regrets. When directions are followed, good things should result.

Substitutions should not be made unless the formula in question lists alternative ingredients. Ad-libbing could be irritating, in more ways than one.

COSMETICS AND THE LAW

Consumers take it for granted that the cosmetics they buy and use are harmless. Considering the number of individual ingredients in a wardrobe of cosmetics and the interaction of one ingredient with another, the possibilities for adverse effects could be multitudinous. The fact that they are not stems from existing laws regulating the manufacture and sale of cosmetics and from the responsibility manufacturers have taken upon themselves to produce and distribute only safe products.

The Federal Food, Drug, and Cosmetic Act went into effect in 1938. In the years since, sales of cosmetics have quadrupled, partly from the fact that consumers have learned to trust in their safety.

Two important aspects of the law concern the safety of the products and the labels and claims manufacturers attach to them.

The act specifically regulates against adulterated cosmetics, those which contain poisonous or deleterious substances which *may* render them injurious to users under conditions prescribed in labeling *or* usual conditions of use. This simply means that if an injury results from a product used in a way never intended by the manufacturer or in a way that is unusual, resulting injuries cannot be blamed upon the manufacturer or distributor of that cosmetic.

The whole idea of the law, it seems, is one of determining the *likelihood* to injure and regulating against *possible* injury. As noted, even if a cosmetic causes discomfort or injury on the part of isolated individuals, it may be judged safe for general use.

Does all this mean that the cosmetics we buy and use are entirely free of poisonous or deleterious ingredients? It does not. *Use* of these substances is not prohibited, only use in sufficient amount or in a way to cause injury to the general public.

Before enactment of the law's provisions, some man-

ufacturers indulged in misleading advertising and labeling, even to the point of making patently outrageous
claims about the benefits of their products.

Women may remember the "nourishing" creams ad-
vertised years ago, creams that were supposed to "feed"
the skin. Noting that the skin does not "eat," authorities
under the federal law forced manufacturers to discontinue
their misleading labeling and advertising. Many such
claims were attacked under the new law.

In the years before enactment, there was understand-
able skepticism about cosmetics and about the wonders
they were supposed to work. Women who bought "miracle"
creams and expected to be wrinkle free in forty-eight
hours were more than a little dismayed to find, after the
prescribed number of hours had passed, that they pos-
sessed the same old wrinkles in the same old places.

During those first few years after enactment, seventy-
two cosmetics faced action under the new regulations.
However, in the past two decades there have been few
such cases, and, from 1950 to 1970, something like nine
cosmetics were seized.

Cosmetic safety is something to keep in mind,
whether you are buying or making preparations. Commercial manufacturers have done an excellent job of
determining product safety before putting their wares on
the market. Consumer trust in modern-day products is,
for the most part, well placed.

5

Basic Instructions for Formulating Cosmetics in the Kitchen

Before beginning to make any cosmetic formula, be certain to read the directions carefully and to assemble all necessary equipment and ingredients. As is true in baking a cake from scratch, the most efficient method of getting all the good things together in a perfect mixture is to be well organized and to know what is happening next.

EQUIPMENT

1. Glass or stainless steel mixing bowls or chemistry beakers. (Beakers are especially handy to work with and are available at hobby shops as well as chemical supply houses. See Appendix B)

25

2. Stainless steel or enameled cookware for heating, including at least one deep double boiler. (A double boiler can be any container suspended over hot water.)

3. Metal candy or laboratory thermometer

4. Eye dropper

5. Measuring cups for dry and for liquid measure

6. At least one set of metal measuring spoons

7. Egg beater

8. Narrow metal spatulas

9. Mortar and pestle. (Sets are available at some drugstores and also from chemical supply houses. Health food stores sometimes carry them. A heavy bowl and wooden "stocking darner" can serve as a substitute.)

10. A piece of frosted or plate glass to be used for working pigments into lipsticks, makeup, etc. (A cheap picture frame from the dime store is one way to buy your glass.)

11. Litmus papers. (Available from hobby and toy shops that sell chemistry sets.)

BUYING INGREDIENTS

The drugstore is the place to begin. Simpler formulas in this volume use materials you can buy today from your druggist. For more complex formulas you will want to order some of the good new things now available for cosmetics. Here again, your druggist can be extremely helpful. He can order specific products from the supplier in reasonable amounts. If your prefer, however, you may write directly to the manufacturer or distributor and tell him what you need and how much you want to buy. Appendix B lists addresses of suppliers.

Health food stores carry most of the oils used in these formulas: avocado, sesame, wheat-germ, and the like. Expect to be surprised by the number of things you will find in your local stores. Many of them have on hand most of the materials called for in this book.

Most ingredients are surprisingly inexpensive. For items not on the drugstore shelf which you may wish to order, consult with the druggist about cost. He should have supply catalogs and price lists available. If you write directly to the source, ask for "small lot" price lists.

MEASURING

The process of measuring ingredients has been simplified to eliminate the need for sophisticated laboratory equipment. All amounts have been converted to measurements familiar to American households—measuring cups and spoons. Measurement conversion is a complicated process, so in the event you uncover an exciting new formula, you had better uncover a chemist as well to help you convert it. Knowledge of the specific gravity (or density) of all ingredients is necessary before beginning the mathematical steps that will tell you how to go from percentages by weight or specified metric measurements to measuring spoons.

Liquids should be measured in glass measuring cups with pouring spouts for full- or partial-cup measurements. Smaller amounts are, of course, measured in your spoons. When making a liquid measurement, hold the measuring cup at eye level to make certain that the liquid is indeed at the proper level.

Dry and very sticky materials should be measured in dry-cup measures (or spoons). A rubber or stainless steel spatula is a convenient tool for emptying materials from cups or spoons to mixing containers.

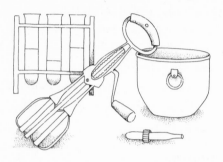

What about waxes? Some waxes come in cakes, others are finely shredded, and still others arrive in large chunks. Beeswax is frequently packaged in 1-ounce cakes and some formulas handily call for just this amount. However, when you need a teaspoon of a solid wax, we suggest using your kitchen grater in measuring. Simply grate the wax as you would a block of Cheddar cheese, then take the pencil-shaving-sized pieces of wax and press them firmly into your metal measure. Just as is true in measuring brown sugar, waxes must be packed tightly so that you are certain you have the right amount. It is an easy and neat process.

Another way to measure waxes (and other ingredients such as thymol or menthyl chunks or flakes) is to put these materials in a beaker and place over water until the wax is melted. Then pour the liquid into the measuring spoon or cup.

HEATING

It is always best to heat ingredients over water; however, in the event that something is to be brought to a boil you may use direct heat—carefully. You may wish to fashion a handy do-it-yourself double boiler for cosmetic concocting. In the author's kitchen, an old Danish coffee pot, tall and narrow, is just right for holding a 600-milliliter beaker over water. And a new metal teakettle has a top that is just right for holding a 400-milliliter beaker. Voila! We have two double boilers that are, by virtue of a heritage part chemistry laboratory and part hardware store, perfect for kitchen cosmeticology.

Double boilers, whatever style, should be narrow and deep. Shallow pans, when you are working with small amounts, make it difficult to mix properly and to determine accurate temperatures.

When instructions indicate that ingredients should be heated to a specific temperature before mixing, believe them. Temperature is important in "putting it all together."

MIXING

Many of the formulas in this book are emulsions—suspensions of oil and water, two ingredients we have always heard were incompatible. Using the right ingredients and the right techniques, the oil part of the formula and the water part are beautifully compatible, forming a delicious-looking snowy emulsion. Emulsifying agents make it all possible by permitting small droplets of oil to remain suspended in water (oil/water emulsions) or small droplets of water to remain suspended in oil (water/oil emulsions).

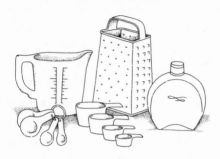

In making these creams, oil and water components are heated separately to a specified temperature. When the correct temperature is reached, one is poured into the other. It is necessary to stir while pouring. Instructions will say to continue stirring until the material cools to a specified temperature, when you may add perfume. Further stirring as the material cools causes it to reach the desired temperature and consistency. Sometimes vigorous stirring is required, in which case the use of an egg beater is ideal.

Not all formulas require heating and cooling. There are many that are simple mixtures of ingredients (such as glycerin and rose water).

Mixing powders and pastes is accomplished in a mortar using a simple rubbing (or grinding) process. In mixing pigments, materials are worked back and forth on a glass plate with a metal spatula. By spreading the base in such a manner it is a simple chore to determine when mixing is complete and the preparation is smooth and even.

In all cases, formula directions for mixing are complete and simple to follow.

USING A THERMOMETER

Using a kitchen or laboratory thermometer properly is an easy procedure—and an important one. Insert the thermometer into heated material, making certain the bulb is completely covered and that it does not touch the container. Read the temperature on the scale, allowing enough time for the thermometer to register the temperature of the material.

Temperature is sometimes a factor in packaging your products. Directions will tell you whether it is necessary to cool a product completely before putting it into a jar, whether it may be poured warm, or whether it should be allowed to stand overnight before packaging. For simple mixtures of ingredients where heating and cooling are not necessary, preparations may be packaged right away.

Temperature measurement can vary with altitude and atmospheric conditions. It is a good idea to calibrate your thermometer so that you will know the readings you are getting are accurate. It is a simple process.

To calibrate your thermometer, test it in water using the boiling point of water as a check to determine how far off the thermometer is. For example, if your thermometer registers 210°F rather than 212°F when the water boils, read your thermometer at two degrees lower than it actually shows. Thus, if you are heating some ingredients to 167°F, when *your* thermometer reads 165°F, that is the temperature you are seeking.

It is a good idea to write yourself a note indicating any such variance between your thermometer and standard readings so you won't forget to make that adjustment when making your cosmetics. A simple written reminder clipped to a page of this volume will serve to keep the need for correction in mind. All you need do is tell yourself "subtract 2°F from all temperatures given in these formulas."

PACKAGING PREPARATIONS

Always use clean containers for your products. There is a world of wonderful ways to package the good things that come from your kitchen—in pots and jars and bottles of every imaginable size and shape. Glass, porcelain, enameled or *glazed* pottery containers work very well for cosmetics.

Think about buying several matched sets of containers when you are planning to brew up some cosmetics for gifts. Use glass paints to decorate the containers, perhaps with the name or initials of the person to whom the gift is going. Individuality is the key.

Instructions with each formula tell you how to package, if directions are needed.

Have fun!

6

Perfumes, Colors, and Preservatives

A red pigment made from henna decorated Egyptian nails, hair, palms, and soles, while red ocher brightened smiles of the ladies of the Nile. Perfumes made from rose and sandalwood enchanted the nostrils and the attention of their gentlemen friends.

Colors and perfumes have been, since the beginning of woman's desire to pique man's desire, of utmost importance in cosmetics. Those who make cosmetics at home need to know how to use these psychologically important ingredients. Too, kitchen cosmeticologists need to understand the basics of preserving the preparations they make, and to know when it is necessary and when it is not.

Fortunately, coloring, perfuming, and preserving good cosmetics are far simpler processes, and far more interesting, in today's kitchen than they were in yester-day's shop along the Nile.

PERFUMES

Today, those who formulate cosmetics commercially recognize the importance of perfumes. They acknowledge that adding fragrance to their preparations makes them more pleasant for the consumers who use them. A very practical aspect of perfuming is that unpleasant odors of basic materials must be masked in order to make the final product acceptable.

Psychological effects of perfume in cosmetics have been evaluated with some rather surprising results. A study has revealed that consumers not only prefer a pleasantly perfumed product, but also link the fragrance of a product with its "perceived quality." A cosmetic product was tested twice in a controlled experiment reported in a professional cosmetics journal. The second time around, the only change in the product was that the perfume was improved. And in that second test, consumers noted all kinds of dramatic improvements in the effectiveness of the preparation. There was no denying the psychological effect of the better perfume.

An important aspect of using perfumes is that of aesthetic compatibility. The kind of perfume used should suit the nature of the product. Woodsy-scented shampoos frequently suggest the out-of-doors, making us feel fresh and clean before we have even begun to wash our hair. But how inappropriate that out-of-doors scent would be behind our ears when we are off for an elegant evening on the town!

There have been all sorts of studies (some conducted by manufacturers who sample consumers' preferences) to determine just what perfume is best for what product. This is particularly important in light of the consumer's attitude about high quality being directly related to fragrance.

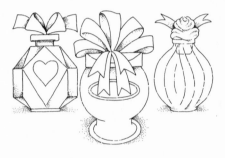

The druggist generally has on hand a variety of perfumes for cosmetic use: for example, rose soluble and bay rum are usually available as are the interesting orange, lemon, lime, and peppermint oils. Remember that perfumes and flavorings used in cosmetics are concentrated especially for this purpose. If you choose to use your personal stock of perfumes, count on using a substantial amount.

The amount of perfume to use in a formulation depends upon the kind of perfume you are working with—whether it is a concentrate or whether it is already diluted. The amount also depends on personal preference. Always use a bit less than you think you will want, then drop in more until your nose is satisfied. The "sniff test" is the best possible means of determining the just-right amount.

Perfume is added for aesthetic value. You may prefer to exclude it from some or all of your preparations.

COLORS

Can you use food coloring in cosmetics? For face and hand creams, shaving preparations, clear lotions, and bath products, a few drops of food coloring, well blended, can give a pleasing effect. *Don't* try food colorings for those cosmetics that require pigments: lipsticks, face powders, makeup, and eye preparations.

Cosmetic pigments are under strict governmental control. All *organic colorants* used in cosmetics are produced according to U.S. Government specifications and are certified for use in drugs and cosmetics by the Food and Drug Administration. They are labeled *D & C certified colorants*. These may *not* be used in foods, and they may *not* be used in products applied to the area of the eye. They *may* be used in lipstick, rouge, face powder, nail lacquer, and liquid makeup.

Inorganic colorants are provisionally approved and listed by the Food and Drug Administration for use in cosmetics, although they are not subject to certification per se. They *may* be used in the cosmetic applications named above, plus they *may* be used in eye preparations. Inorganic colorants do not carry a D & C color number—D & C Red #21—but rather a designation—Cosmetic Brown.

Always request a manufacturer's color chart when

you order pigments so that you will know for certain that the colorant you are using is right for the preparation you have in mind. It's not nearly as complicated as it sounds, and the chart will make the whole process simple, besides, the chart, with it's "paint chips," is a marvelous help in deciding which colorants you want to use.

Coloring instructions for rouge, lipstick, face powders, eye preparations, and makeup are given with the individual formulas. A general rule of thumb is to *go lightly*—a pinch of color will turn a cream makeup from white to a light golden tan.

In coloring makeup, you may wish to put on your mixing glass a dab of commercially made product you are now using, then work toward matching (or not matching) it. Blending pigments is one of the most exciting, and most satisfying, aspects of cosmetic making.

Experiment with both colors and fragrances, keeping in mind the physical and the psychological aspects of this phase of creating cosmetics.

Appropriateness is the key. Can you imagine the reaction to a rose-scented, pale pink after-shave lotion?

PRESERVATIVES

Most commercially made cosmetics, which may reach you months after manufacture, contain preservatives to keep them from spoiling. Do you need to preserve yours?

It depends. When you make a preparation for your own use, it is safe to assume that you will have used it before there is any need to worry about spoilage. Most of these preparations will last a month or more without spoiling. Of course if they are kept in the refrigerator, they will last much longer. One of the advantages of making your own cosmetics is that you make them fresh and use them fresh. You shouldn't need to worry about preservatives under these conditions. And, if a product is likely to spoil in a relatively short time, a note on the formula advises you that such is the case and suggests adding a preservative.

Gift cosmetics that you fear might not be used right away may be labeled "keep under refrigeration" or may be made with preservatives added.

A professional, general-purpose preservative for cosmetics is this: dissolve 1/4 teaspoon of methyl para-hydroxybenzoate (called, more simply, "methyl paraben") in 2 teaspoons of ethyl alcohol. Add 1/4 teaspoon of this solution to the non-oily or non-waxy portion of the formula when you are making it.

Methyl paraben can be ordered through your druggist, but make certain you give him the full name.

Or you may substitute the following:

For eye preparations, add a pinch of boric acid. For creams and preparations that are *non-acidic* (basic cold creams, the lubricating cream, etc.), add a few drops of white tincture of iodine to the non-oil or non-wax portion of the formula before heating. For creams or other preparations that are *acidic*, add a pinch of salicylic acid to the oil portion of the formula. For formulas whose major ingredient is water, add a pinch of boric acid. Preparations already containing boric acid need no further preservative.

Now, if you want to use one of these methods of preserving and you are uncertain about the acidity of the preparation involved, use litmus paper (available at hobby shops) on a trial batch to determine the answer. You'll want to make the formula once for yourself before making it for a gift in any event, so this shouldn't constitute an extra step. Lay a strip of litmus on top of a cream or creamy lotion, or dip the strip into a clear lotion. If the preparation is acidic, it will turn blue litmus red; if it is basic, it will turn red litmus blue.

You probably will not need to concern yourself very much with preservatives. Remember the "keep under refrigeration" label for your gifts—it might be the easiest answer!

7

Caring for the Skin

Most authorities interested in such matters credit a second-century Roman physician, Claudius Galenus, with making the first cold cream. Others insist that Hippocrates concocted the first cold cream centuries earlier.

Galenus' directions for making the cream appeared in his *Methodus Medendi vel de Morbis Curandis,* where he notes that one part of purified wax is carefully liquefied in a mortar together with three or four parts of olive oil (in which rose petals have been macerated) and then allowed to cool, whereupon as much water as can be incorporated in the above mass is added.

Another early cold cream formula was recorded in the *Pharmacopoeia Collegii Regalis Medicorum Londinensis* of 1617, under the name *Unquentum Refrigerans.*

By whatever name and in whatever era, creams have

been used to treat the skin: to cleanse, lubricate, soften, and protect the body's covering. And the traditional cream, since who-knows-when, has been cold cream.

Why are cold creams called cold?

A true cold cream has a relatively large amount of water in its formula. When the cream is applied, the emulsion breaks down, and, when the water evaporates, a cooling sensation is produced on the skin.

Cold creams are often referred to as the basic creams or all purpose creams. Variations in formulas make them more or less versatile, but in general they can be considered the mainstay of cosmetic creams. They are used for cleansing, softening, lubricating, and making a woman feel a lot better and more relaxed than before she used them. There is an undeniable boost to the morale, a mental and physical feeling of being refreshed, when cooling creams are applied to the skin.

Surely the greatest problem of caring for the skin is keeping it clean and functioning properly, a problem compounded in this modern age by an urban atmosphere permeated with a variety of pollutants unknown to Galenus. In order for a skin to retain its health it must be cleansed thoroughly and regularly and treated with preparations to help it keep its tone and beauty through the years.

No doubt someone you know has a favorite story about a woman who, to care for her skin, used *only* pure soap and water, or glycerin and rose water, or olive oil and salt, or cucumber juice, or lemon-scented cold cream, and who lived to be ninety-seven and was wrinkle free the whole distance.

It is true that skin condition can be unusually fine in a person of advanced age, but there is probably very little truth in stories of the magic worked by *one* special preparation used for a lifetime. There are many factors in keeping a skin lovely and healthy, and the preparations used on it are only part of the answer. Diet and general health, to name two other factors, are important.

A good routine for skin care includes using a mask a couple of times weekly for cleansing and toning the skin. It includes *always* creaming off makeup before retiring, and using a good lubricant on the skin at night. If you share your bed with a man who objects to sleeping next to a greasy face, then use a dry-skin vanishing cream. He'll never know.

Your skin care routine should include the use of a vanishing or foundation cream under makeup.

It should include giving your face a gentle massage when you apply a lubricating cream—it feels wonderful and stimulates the skin. Work *up and out* on the cheeks, and don't forget to smooth creams *upward* on the neck.

The skin should be cleansed regularly, and, if a soap is preferred for cleansing, it is more important than ever that a lubricating cream be added to the regular beauty routine. Most women seem to prefer using a cream or lotion for cleansing because this method *feels* better than using soap. Cosmetic creams and lotions are excellent cleansers and are, with apologies to soap advocates, more effective than soap. If you doubt this, try using a good cleansing cream after a soap and water attack on makeup and grime. You'll find the evidence on the tissue.

Some realities about skin care you might think about

are these: *no* externally applied preparation is going to make those lines around your eyes disappear, although use of a good lubricating cream can lessen the problem and can *delay* aging; similarly, *no* externally applied preparation is going to cure dry skin, but the application of suitable creams can alleviate the symptoms and keep the skin soft, hydrated, and oiled.

It must be remembered that skin needs protection from the elements. Sun and wind can burn and chafe, and a dry climate can mean a dry skin. Creams fight the elements and can help you put your best face forward in spite of wind and weather.

Remember too, that skin care shouldn't stop at the neck. Elbows, knees and, especially, the feet need some kind, gentle softening now and then with a good cream or lotion. And if you are going to be spending some time out of doors during the summer, make use of an oil or lotion with a good sunscreen in it.

Caring for the skin means all-over body care. While our faces seem to be most important and seem to demand our attention each time we look into a mirror, we must remember that there are lots of square inches of pretty body-covering we need to take care of.

Most women use a collection of face creams—cold, cleansing, lubricating, vanishing—while others rely on one or two, perhaps a good basic cold cream and a rich lubricating cream. It all depends on personal preference and needs.

Among the skin care products that women enjoy and that can be made successfully at home are these:

CREAMS

COLD CREAMS (discussed above) are all-purpose creams used for both cleansing and lubricating. They are basically water-in-oil creams (greasy) or oil-in-water (non-greasy) creams. They have a pleasant, softening effect on the skin.

CLEANSING CREAMS may be simple cold creams or more complex formulas. Their job is to penetrate the fine crevices of the skin and to dissolve foreign particles hidden there. They serve to get rid of accumulated grime and makeup. The lotion form is an emulsion made of lighter oils held in suspension in water, which means that it does its work without leaving a greasy feeling.

VANISHING CREAMS are so called because they seem to disappear into the skin, leaving no trace of grease or oil. They do leave a protective film on the skin, however. Some recent formulas for vanishing creams include lanolin, and frequently other ingredients are added to modify the soap base of the preparations.

LUBRICATING CREAMS are frequently rich in lanolin, the substance extracted from wool that effectively serves as a substitute for natural oils of the skin. A lubricating cream has its basis in a cold cream, but with the addition of lanolin becomes effective in treating the skin for dryness. Consistent use of a good lubricating cream means the skin not only fights drying but also becomes softer and more pliant.

ASTRINGENT LOTIONS are sometimes recommended to close the pores before makeup application or to minimize problems with enlarged pores. It is true that their application seems to make such pore openings less conspicuous; however, the openings affected are not pores but the openings of hair follicles.

The lotions have a delightfully refreshing feeling and are especially pleasing when used during hot, sticky weather. Aromatic waters, such as rose and orange flower, are often used for their aesthetic value in astringent lotions.

Even if they aren't attacking enlarged pores, astringent lotions are pleasing to use and leave the face feeling tingly and alive. And that is saying a lot for a cosmetic.

What are astringent lotions? Actually, they are very mild anti-perspirants.

MASKS

Masks were used not only by Cleopatra, but undoubtedly by her great-grandmother, for masks (or packs) have been used to cleanse and tone the skin since earliest antiquity. Interestingly, they are now increasing in popularity, and one reason for their being so strongly in vogue may be the unfortunate influence of air pollutants. Another reason is the combination of physical and psychological stimulation that comes from the effects of a mask, with its warming and tightening of the skin plus thorough cleansing.

The tightening effect of a mask is produced by its drying. Surface active materials work during drying to remove impurities from the skin, and the result, when the hardened mask is washed away, is a tingling, fresh, and gleaming skin. Many women use a mask several times a week; others only when they want to look especially lovely. Frequent use should not harm the skin in any way, but should serve to help it keep its tone just that much longer.

HAND CREAMS AND LOTIONS

"Which pair of hands is 17 years old and which is 35?" asks a magazine advertisement. Too often, for most women, there is no contest, for hands show age very quickly. While any skin surface will withstand the moderate use of soap and water for an indefinite period of time, there is usually nothing very moderate about the continued exposure to soap and water suffered by a woman's hands. If care is not taken to replace oils lost in that exposure, rough red skin results which can lead not only to a beauty problem but also to a health problem.

The skin secretes a natural lubricant, sebum, which serves to keep it healthy. When sebum is lost more rapidly than it is normally produced, the skin loses its pliability and becomes dry and scaly. To compound the problem of "kitchen hands," breaks appear in the skin surface which give bacteria a chance to invade and cause infection.

The function of a hand cream or lotion is to keep the outer layer of skin soft, pliable, and healthy and to prevent cracking of surface skin.

POWDERS

Body powders are among the oldest cosmetics. For centuries men and women have dusted their bodies with lightly scented powders and have sprinkled mild powders on their infants. Body powders soothe and protect the skin; they reduce the chance of irritation to the body's covering.

Good absorbent properties are a must in talcum and baby powders. Softness and slip (the ability of particles to slide easily) are also important properties.

The most commonly used material in these powders is talc. Other ingredients are added to improve absorption, adhesive qualities, and texture.

TANNING PREPARATIONS

A sun-bronzed skin is appealing to most of us, usually because a golden tan enhances a person's looks and gives the impression of an outdoorsy, healthful kind of existence. And when we think of a sun tan as being healthy, we are, in part, correct, for sunshine supplies our bodies with vitamin D. The problem comes from too much exposure to the sun at one time or continued exposure without proper care of the skin during those hours outdoors.

The increased popularity of the golden tan has been

responsible for a world of products that promise to protect from burn, enhance tanning (with or without the sun), and soothe and protect the skin. It is the wise person at the pool who takes along—and uses—a good sunscreen and tanning agent. A chemical sunscreen is needed to allow only the tanning rays to work on the skin. It is the difference between looking good and suffering the torment of scorched skin.

Products that screen out the harmful rays of the sun and permit the beneficial, tanning rays to come through have been developed by physicists, dermatologists, and chemists working as a team using combined knowledge of light, the skin, and chemistry.

A good sun tan preparation that will protect and provide desired tanning results is one of the simplest cosmetics to make and one of the least expensive. It is an extremely satisfactory homemade product.

CREAMS

Basic Cold Cream No. 1

One of the most common cosmetic emollients used by women is a basic cold cream. It is considered to be the most important facial cream used. This type of cream contains mineral oil and wax which are emulsified in water with a small amount of borax. This formula is typical of the kind of cream women rely on to serve many purposes such as cleansing, lubricating, and softening.

Mineral oil	*1/2 cup*
Beeswax	*1-ounce block or 2 tablespoons plus 1 teaspoon*
Borax	*2/3 of 1/4 teaspoon **
Distilled water	*1/4 cup plus 1 teaspoon*
Perfume, as desired	

Heat the mineral oil and beeswax in the top of a double boiler. The water in the outer pot should be brought to a boil and the wax should be thoroughly melted. In a separate pan, dissolve the borax in the water and bring to a boil. Add this in a thin stream to the melted wax, while stirring vigorously in one direction. When temperature drops to 140°F (60°C), add 1 teaspoon perfume oil, if desired, and continue stirring until the temperature drops to 120°F (49°C). At this point, pour into jars. *Yield: 1 cup.*

Basic Cold Cream No. 2

A variation on Basic Cold Cream No. 1, this cream is softer and smoother. Those who prefer a stiffer cream should stick to formula No. 1; those who enjoy a softer, fluffier cream will prefer formula No. 2.

Mineral oil	*1/2 cup plus 1 tablespoon*
Beeswax	*1-ounce block or 2 tablespoons plus 1 teaspoon*
Borax	*1/4 teaspoon*
Distilled water	*1/4 cup plus 1 tablespoon*
Perfume, as desired	

* Pour 1/4 level teaspoon of borax on a piece of clean paper. Using a table knife, divide the borax into three parts, discarding one part and using the 2/3 for your cream. (One-fourth teaspoon really isn't as minute as it sounds, and dividing it this way is a simple process.)

Heat mineral oil and beeswax in top of double boiler to 158°F (70°C). In the top of a second double boiler dissolve borax in water and heat to same temperature. Add water and borax to melted wax slowly, while stirring. Stir until cream cools to 113–122°F (45–50°C). Add 1 teaspoon perfume and stir until perfume is evenly dispersed. When temperature drops to 120°F (49°C), pour into jars. *Yield: 1 cup.*

Basic Cold Cream No. 3

Addition of paraffin wax in this formula creates the smoothest of this series of basic cold creams. The appearance (but fortunately not the consistency) resembles whipped marshmallow cream. It is also the least greasy of the creams.

Borax	*1/4 teaspoon*
Mineral oil	*1/3 cup plus 1 tablespoon plus 2 teaspoons*
Beeswax	*1-ounce block or 2 tablespoons plus 1 teaspoon*
Paraffin wax	*2 3/4 teaspoons*
Distilled water	*1/4 cup plus 1 1/2 teaspoons*
Perfume, as desired	

Dissolve borax in water, heat in top of double boiler to 167°F (75°C). Heat waxes and oil in a second double boiler to 158°F (70°C). Add the oil and wax mixture *to the water solution,* with vigorous stirring. Continue to stir until mixture cools to 122°F (50°C), and add perfume if desired. *Yield: 1 cup.*

Theatrical Cold Cream

This traditional formula is especially suited to cleansing and softening skins to which heavy makeup has been applied. It makes an unusual gift for friends who are Little Theater buffs.

Mineral oil	*1/2 cup plus 1/2 teaspoon*
Synthetic spermaceti wax	*1 tablespoon plus 1/4 teaspoon*
Beeswax	*2 tablespoons plus 1 3/4 teaspoons*
Borax	*1 3/4 teaspoons*
Distilled water	*1/4 cup plus 2 tablespoons*
Perfume, as desired	

Heat mineral oil, spermaceti wax, and beeswax in the top of double boiler until it reaches a temperature of 160°F (72°C). Dissolve borax in water and heat to same temperature. Slowly add the water/borax solution to the wax mixture. Beat slowly until the entire mixture reaches a temperature of 122°F (50°C). Let stand and stir occasionally until temperature falls to 110°F (43°C). Add perfume to suit. Stir occasionally until temperature reaches 104°F (40°C), then pour into jars. *Yield: 1 1/4 cups.*

All-Purpose Cream

This all-purpose cream softens and lubricates the skin. It is a delicious-looking and delicious-feeling cream, a smooth treat for tired skin.

Mineral oil	*1/4 cup*
Beeswax	*2 teaspoons*
Arlacel 83	*1/4 teaspoon*
Lanolin	*3/4 teaspoon*
Borax	*1/8 teaspoon*
Distilled water	*2 tablespoons plus 1 teaspoon*
Perfume, as desired	

Heat mineral oil, beeswax, Arlacel 83, and lanolin in the top of a double boiler to 158–167°F (70–75°C). Dissolve borax in water and heat in another double boiler to 167°F (75°C). Add borax/water solution to mineral oil mixture gradually while stirring. Whip with vigor until combined mixture reaches 131–140°F (55–60°C). Perfume and pour into jar. *Yield: 1/2 cup.*

Cleansing Cream No. 1

The water content in this unusually soft cleansing cream results in a smoother consistency than is found in many other products of this nature, and it increases the effectiveness of the preparation in cleaning away water-soluble grime. It is an extremely effective cleanser—witness the results when you tissue off dirt and makeup.

Mineral oil	*3 tablespoons plus 2 teaspoons*
Beeswax	*1 1/4 teaspoons*
Synthetic spermaceti wax	*1 1/4 teaspoons*
Lanolin	*1/4 teaspoon*
Distilled water	*2 tablespoons plus 1 1/2 teaspoons*
Perfume, as desired	

Measure mineral oil into top of double boiler. Add beeswax, spermaceti, and lanolin. Heat until mixture is smooth and clear. Slowly pour in heated distilled water, stirring constantly. Continue stirring until mixture drops to 104°F (40°C); add perfume to suit. Stir until mixture reaches 86°F (30°C), then pour into jar. *Yield: 1/2 cup.*

Cleansing Cream No. 2

Here is another efficient cleansing cream, one which works well at removing makeup and grime from the face. It is a stiffer cream than the Cleansing Cream No. 1 formula produces. Try them both to see which you prefer.

Paraffin wax	*1 1/4 teaspoons*
Beeswax	*2 1/2 teaspoons*
Mineral oil	*1/4 cup plus 1/2 teaspoon*
Stearic acid	*1/4 teaspoon*
Boric acid	*1/8 teaspoon*
Distilled water	*1 tablespoon plus 2 teaspoons*
Perfume, as desired	

Heat paraffin, beeswax, mineral oil, and stearic acid in top of double boiler to 158°F (70°C). Dissolve boric acid in water and heat in second double boiler to the same temperature. Add the boric acid/water solution to the wax mixture slowly, while stirring. Continue stirring until the mixture reaches 113–122°F (45–50°C). Add perfume, stirring continuously, and pour as mixture begins to thicken.

Don't panic when you first add the boric acid/water solution to the waxes. At first it looks as if they are not going to mix, but, with vigorous stirring during cooling, they will. *Yield: 1/2 cup.*

Liquid Cleansing Cream

A light, delightful, and efficient cleanser, this liquid cosmetic is simple to make and is similar to those that are current best sellers on the cosmetic market.

Mineral oil	*1/2 cup plus 1 teaspoon*
Beeswax	*1 teaspoon*
Span 60	*1 teaspoon*
Tween 60	*1 1/2 teaspoons*
G-2162	*1 tablespoon*
Distilled water	*1 cup plus 1 1/2 teaspoons*
Perfume, *as desired*	

Heat all ingredients *except water* in top of double boiler to a temperature of 158°F (70°C). Heat distilled water to same temperature and add to the oil and wax mixture. Beat very slowly until thoroughly mixed. Add perfume at 104°F (40°C), and bottle. *Yield: 1 1/2 cups.*

Cleansing Lotion

A marvelous, clear product that refreshes while cleansing. It is an especially easy formula, with all ingredients as close as the drug store. Use a few drops of food coloring to make the product look as beautiful as it is!

Borax	*1/8 teaspoon*
Distilled water	*1/4 cup plus 2 teaspoons*
Witch hazel	*2 1/2 teaspoons*
Denatured *ethyl alcohol*	*1 tablespoon plus 2 teaspoons*

Dissolve borax in water (heat if necessary). Cool then add other ingredients.   *Yield: 1/2 cup.*

Cleansing Milk

Under various intriguing titles such as *laits virginals* or *laits de beauté,* complexion milks have been used for many, many years. In fact, the idea of bathing in milk itself has been in and out of popularity over the centuries.

Modern milks are essentially diluted cleansing creams that have the appearance of milk. They are pleasing products to use, and retain something of the romance of their history. They are quite good at getting into lines and creases in the skin (never say wrinkles) to do their cleansing job.

Mineral oil	*2 1/2 teaspoons*
Cetyl alcohol *(1-hexadecanol)*	*1/8 teaspoon*
Stearic acid	*3/4 teaspoon*
Triethanolamine	*scant 1/2 teaspoon*
Distilled water	*1/3 cup plus 1 teaspoon*
Perfume, *as desired*	

Heat mineral oil, cetyl alcohol, and stearic acid in top of double boiler to 158°F (70°C). Heat triethanolamine and water to the same temperature in a second double boiler. Add water solution to the oil mixture slowly, while stirring. Continue to stir until the mixture reaches 104–113°F (40–45°C) and add perfume. Continue stirring until the mixture drops to 77°F (25°C) and pour into bottle.   *Yield: 1/2 cup.*

Simple Vanishing Cream

Vanishing creams are non-greasy soapy creams which leave a thin, protective film on the skin, even though they seem to "vanish" after application. They are sometimes used as a powder base.

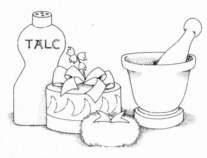

Be patient when making this particular cream, for at first, it has the look of soapy dishwater. Then, as you stir and it cools, it becomes one of the most beautiful, snowy creams imaginable. It is an extremely satisfactory product.

Stearic acid	*1/4 cup plus 3 tablespoons*
Potassium carbonate	*1/2 teaspoon*
Glycerin	*2 tablespoons plus 2 teaspoons*
Distilled water	*1 cup plus 1 tablespoon*
Perfume,	
as desired	

Stearic acid is a powder which melts when heated. Place it in the top of a double boiler, and melt over hot water. Measure the potassium carbonate, glycerin, and water into another pan and heat *just* to a boil. Pour the water solution into the melted stearic acid slowly, in a thin stream, stirring vigorously while pouring. When all the water solution has been added, stir slowly with spatula until the carbon dioxide bubbles stop rising. Then you may remove the top of the double boiler from the heat and continue stirring. When the cream has reached 135°F (57°C), add perfume oil and blend in well. Continue stirring from time to time until the cream is cool. Let stand for several hours before a final stirring. Then pack into a container. *Yield: 1 1/4 cups.*

Dry-Skin Vanishing Cream

This vanishing cream has a high lanolin content to help fight dry skin problems. As do all vanishing creams, it leaves a protective film on the skin that is invisible. This product looks something like a puff of whipped cream when you are first working with it. A luscious, efficient cosmetic, it is guaranteed to delight dry skin.

Lanolin	*2 teaspoons*
Stearic acid	*3 tablespoons plus 1 1/2 teaspoons*
Triethanolamine	*1/2 teaspoon*
Distilled water	*1/2 cup plus 1/2 teaspoon*
Diethylene glycol monoethyl ether	*1 tablespoon plus 1 teaspoon*
Perfume, as desired	

Heat lanolin and stearic acid in top of double boiler to a temperature of 185°F (85°C). Over low flame, heat triethanolamine, water, and diethylene glycol monoethyl ether until the solution reaches the same temperature. Then add the water solution to the mixture in the double boiler, pouring slowly and stirring vigorously. If you have a friend handy to help, use your egg beater to stir while the friend pours the water solution for you. Allow the emulsion to cool, stirring occasionally to avoid any crust formation at the surface. Leave the cream overnight and add perfume the next day. Stir until the cream is soft, then put into jar. After a few days, the cream will stiffen a bit.   *Yield: 3/4 cup.*

Avocado Moisturizer

This is a wonderful beauty preparation which leaves the skin soft and smooth and effectively serves as a moisturizer. It is one of the finest preparations you can make at home, and one of the most pleasing. It is a semi-liquid preparation.

Mineral oil	*2 teaspoons*
Ceresine wax	*1/2 teaspoon*
Isopropyl myristate	*2 tablespoons plus 1 teaspoon*
Almond oil (sweet)	*1 tablespoon plus 1 1/2 teaspoons*
Avocado oil	*1 tablespoon plus 1 1/2 teaspoons*
Lanolin, liquid	*1 tablespoon plus 1 teaspoon*
Perfume, *as desired*	

Put all ingredients in top of double boiler. Melt and blend until mixture is uniform. Remove from heat and continue stirring. Perfume and put in jar.   *Yield: 1/2 cup.*

Lubricating Cream

This is a super-rich lubricating cream that should do wonders for girls eighteen to eighty. It is especially effective if applied at night when it can be left alone to do its work.

Just for fun, the author computed the cost of making this excellent cream—20¢ (a generous estimate). To buy a cream of this quality, one would expect to pay approximately $4, so it seems you not only save face with this cream, but also dollars.

Mineral oil	*2 tablespoons*
Olive oil	*1 teaspoon*
Lanolin	*2 3/4 teaspoons*
Stearic acid	*1 teaspoon*
Synthetic spermaceti wax	*1 1/2 teaspoons*
Cetyl alcohol	*3 1/4 teaspoons*
Triethanolamine	*2 teaspoons*
Distilled water	*2 tablespoons plus 2 teaspoons*
Perfume, as desired	

Heat mineral oil, olive oil, lanolin, stearic acid, spermaceti, and cetyl alcohol in top of double boiler to a temperature of 158°F (70°C). Heat triethanolamine and water to the same temperature and add to first mixture, stirring continuously. Stir to a temperature of 122°F (50°C), then perfume. When perfume is completely blended in, pour cream into jar. *Yield: 1/2 cup.*

SKIN LOTIONS

Astringent Lotion

Astringent lotions act to tighten the skin and are frequently used for their "wake-up" feeling.

Potassium or	
ammonium alum *	*1/2 teaspoon*
Glycerin	*1 teaspoon*
Orange flower water	*2 tablespoons plus 1 teaspoon*
Rose water	*2 tablespoons plus 1 teaspoon*
Distilled water	*1 tablespoon plus 1 teaspoon*

Dissolve alum in distilled water over gentle heat. Add glycerin; stir. When solution is cooled, add the flower waters and blend to a smooth lotion.   *Yield: 1/3 cup.*

Skin Freshener

As its name implies, this preparation freshens the skin, and, as a side effect, refreshes the spirit.

Borax	*1/4 teaspoon*
Alcohol, ethyl	*2 teaspoons*
Rose water	*3 tablespoons*
Distilled water	*3 tablespoons*

Dissolve borax in water over gentle heat. Cool; add alcohol and rose water. Stir until well blended.   *Yield: 1/2 cup.*

MASKS

Kaolin Mask

This is an extremely effective mask and a very simple one to make. It washes off with warm water, leaving the skin feeling fresh and clean.

* You need only ask your druggist for alum.

Kaolin	*1/2 cup*
Tincture of benzoin	*2 teaspoons*
Distilled water	*sufficient*

Measure kaolin into mortar, add tincture of benzoin, and rub down well until the characteristic odor of the tincture disappears. Add the water, slowly. Rub well. Use enough water to make a *runny paste*. Pack in an air-tight container. *Yield: 3/4 cup.*

Gelatin Mask

This thick, liquid mask is pleasant to use and rinses off with warm water. It serves to cleanse and tone the skin. Be certain to keep container *tightly capped* when not in use. Also, this mask needs to be shaken well before use so that it will pour.

Gum tragacanth	*1 teaspoon*
Glycerin	*1/2 teaspoon*
Gelatin	*1 teaspoon*
Distilled water	*1/3 cup plus 1 tablespoon*
Zinc oxide	*1/4 teaspoon*

Moisten the gum tragacanth with half the glycerin. (Add a few *drops* more glycerin if needed to make a runny paste.) Add gelatin to the water and warm in top of double boiler. Stir until gelatin is dissolved, then add to gum tragacanth and stir. Moisten the zinc oxide with the rest of the glycerin and add to the mixture. If lumps form, use an egg beater to blend. The final mixture will be runny when you bottle it. It will thicken overnight—in fact to the point where a vigorous shake is necessary before using.

It is recommended that this mask be warmed before

using, although we have used it as it comes from the bottle. *Yield: 1/2 cup.*

HAND CREAMS AND LOTIONS

Simple Hand Cream (Oily)

This formula from out of the past uses only three, readily available ingredients in its composition. You may wish to add color as well as perfume, for the finished product is not a snowy white but an off white.

Since the cream has over 70 percent oil plus two waxes, you know the finished product has to be oily in texture. For rough, dry hands it is soothing and softening.

Note: this is a good formula to make while watching television, for it takes a while for the congealing to take place. So, find a comfortable chair and be content to stir gently while you are waiting for the temperature to drop and congealing to occur.

Beeswax	*1 tablespoon plus 1 teaspoon*
Synthetic spermaceti wax	*1 tablespoon plus 1 teaspoon*
Almond oil (sweet)	*2/3 cup plus 1 tablespoon plus 1 teaspoon*

Heat beeswax and spermaceti in top of double boiler to 158°F (70°C). Warm almond oil to same temperature and add slowly to waxes while stirring. Remove heat and stir until temperature drops to 104°F (40°C), when you may add perfume. Pour into container at 86°F (30°C). *Yield: 1 cup.*

Glycerin and Rose Water

This is our favorite hand-care product. If possible, it should be used for a few minutes daily to keep cuticles soft and to avoid hangnails.

Distilled water	*1 cup*
Rose oil (*soluble*)	*2 teaspoons*
Glycerin	*1/4 cup plus 1 tablespoon*

Blend all ingredients until smooth and clear.   *Yield: 1 1/3 cups.*

Avocado Cream

Avocado oil is rich in vitamin A, in some B vitamins, and also contains vitamins D and E, linolenic acid, sterols, and lecithin. Its use in cosmetics is traditional.

There has been some technical debate about just *how* valuable avocado oil is in cosmetics and the extent to which it does or does not penetrate. For the consumer, however, there is no doubting that avocado cream is a very satisfactory cosmetic—rich, softening, lubricating. And that, as we have noted, is the test of any cosmetic preparation.

Mineral oil	*2 1/4 teaspoons*
Ceresine wax	*1/2 teaspoon*
Lanolin	*1 tablespoon plus 1 1/2 teaspoons*
Isopropyl myristate	*2 tablespoons plus 1 teaspoon*
Almond oil (*sweet*)	*1 tablespoon plus 1 1/2 teaspoons*
Avocado oil	*1 tablespoon plus 1 1/2 teaspoons*
Perfume, *as desired*	

Heat mineral oil, ceresine, and lanolin, in top of double boiler to 158°F (70°C). Add isopropyl myristate; stir. Add oils and blend thoroughly. Cool to 104°F (40°C) and perfume. While still liquid pour into container and allow to cool to room temperature. *Yield: 1/2 cup.*

Deluxe Hand Cream

A lovely softening cream that disappears into the skin without leaving a greasy feeling. Texture is light and smooth.

Stearic acid	*3 tablespoons*
Mineral oil	*1 1/2 teaspoons*
Arlacel 60	*1 teaspoon*
Tween 60	*2 teaspoons*
Sorbo	*3 tablespoons*
Distilled water	*1/3 cup plus 2 tablespoons*
Preservative *	
Perfume, as desired	

Heat stearic acid, mineral oil, Arlacel 60, and Tween 60 in top of double boiler over water until mixture reaches a temperature of 162°F (72°C). Heat Sorbo, water, and preservative in separate double boiler until it reaches the same temperature. Add the Sorbo solution to the stearic acid mixture. Stir rapidly while pouring. Stir until cream sets; then perfume, and pour into jar. *Yield: 1 cup.*

---

* This cream may tend to spoil before some others. Keep it refrigerated, or preserve according to instructions in "Perfumes, Colors, and Preservatives" on pp. 37–39.

POWDERS

Baby Powder

A soothing powder for baby's tender skin.

Talc	*1/4 cup*
Kaolin	*2 teaspoons*
Boric acid	*1 tablespoon*
Calcium carbonate (precipitated chalk)	*1 teaspoon*
Zinc stearate	*2 teaspoons*
Perfume, as desired	
Color, as desired	

Put all ingredients except for color and perfume into mortar. Rub down well, then add perfume. A few drops of food coloring may be used to tint the powder a delicate color. *Yield: 1/2 cup.*

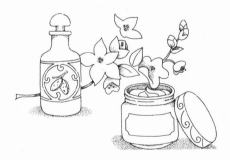

Talcum Powders

Talcum powder is an old-fashioned cosmetic still very much in vogue. It makes an especially nice gift. Follow-

ing are three simple-to-make talcums. Use food coloring
to give them a pretty tint.

TALCUM POWDER NO. 1

Boric acid	*1 1/2 teaspoons*
Talc	*1/4 cup plus 1 tablespoon*
Perfume,	
as desired	

Put powders in mortar and rub well. Add perfume and rub
until well blended.   *Yield: 1/3 cup.*

TALCUM POWDER NO. 2

Boric acid	*2 teaspoons*
Starch (corn,	
rice, potato, etc.)	*3 teaspoons*
Talc	*1/4 cup*
Perfume,	
as desired	

See directions above.   *Yield: 1/3 cup.*

TALCUM POWDER NO. 3

Boric acid	*1 1/2 teaspoons*
Zinc oxide	*1/2 teaspoon*
Starch (corn,	
rice, potato, etc.)	*3 teaspoons*
Talc	*1/4 cup*
Perfume,	
as desired	

See directions above.   *Yield: 1/3 cup.*

TANNING PREPARATIONS

Sun Tan Oil

Preparations designed to keep you from burning and to enhance tanning are basically made of a sun screen, which shuts out the harmful rays of the sun and welcomes tanning rays, and a lubricant which acts as a carrier for the sun screen.

Many sun-worshippers prefer to use a tanning oil. And many are true do-it-yourselfers when it comes to coating the skin with oil, raiding the pantry for olive oil or salad oil in preparation for a stay at the beach. The problem with pantry products is that they lack chemical sun screens.

This simple to make protective oil is an effective and an extremely economical approach to skin care during the summer hours out of doors.

Any pure vegetable oil	*1/2 cup*
Phenyl salicylate crystals	*1 tablespoon*
Color, as desired	
Perfume, as desired	

Shake the oil and crystals together in tightly closed bottle. Add food coloring to create a nice brown tint, then perfume lightly if you wish. *Yield: 1/2 cup.*

Sun Tan Cream

This super-simple tanning cream will appeal to those who enjoy long hours in the sun but who do not enjoy the feel of an oily tanning preparation. It will protect the skin from burning and will enhance tanning, the basic chores of all tanning preparations.

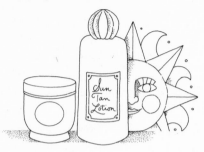

The cold cream called for in this formula may already be a favorite in your cosmetics cabinet, or it may be one of those included in this book.

Basic cold cream	*1/2 cup*
Phenyl salicylate crystals	*1 1/2 tablespoons*
Petrolatum	*1/4 cup*

Dissolve crystals in melted petrolatum. Cool, then blend with cold cream.   *Yield: 3/4 cup.*

8

Hormones and Vitamins

PENETRATING QUESTIONS

Is there truly a fountain of youth? Can its waters be perfumed, poured into cosmetic jars which are elegantly labeled, and then whisked off to our neighborhood stores? And can we buy, you and I, some of this magical stuff to hide the effects of age?

Perhaps. At least in a sense.

The cosmetics most of us buy and use are those intended to protect, cleanse, condition, and decorate the skin and hair. Wise use of these will beautify, and will impede degeneration of the skin due to harmful external forces.

Cosmetic science, not content to rest with its impressive achievements on our behalf, has been for many years experimenting with preparations intended to affect deeper epidermal layers—preparations designed to delay aging and to "plump up" the skin, making it more youthful, more elastic, and more radiant.

One wonders just how much effect our craving for such products has on manufacturers who keep searching for the key to youthful skin. What possibly could be more appealing to a woman in her middle years than the promise of a face that looks ten, or even twenty years younger? Say what you will about growing old gracefully, nobody wants to do it unless she can do it under cover. Americans, in particular, are youth-oriented, and while European men may delight in the older countenances of more mature woman, in this country things don't work that way.

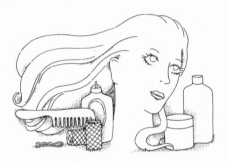

And so our own desires to look young and to radiate health almost force chemists and manufacturers to keep at the job of seeking effective ingredients to rejuvenate our skins. We are waiting, with bated breath and drying skins, for something new.

Because of these feelings, women have been willing to try anything and everything that even implies it will do the job. In years past, many have been disappointed, at times even duped, by cosmetics supposedly able to bring about a younger look.

Now, however, modern chemical research can prove that there are ingredients that will lessen the effects of aging on our skins. And we should learn as much about them as possible.

Since this is a relatively new area of cosmetic research and one which must be handled with great caution, kitchen cosmeticologists are urged not to try brewing up their own magic potions for youth. It is a hazardous area for anyone but the professional cosmetic chemist.

It is not our intent to discuss in detail the physiology of the skin, but in order to understand something of the value of preparations with deep effect, it is necessary to become at least acquainted with what is underneath that pretty face we show the world.

Like all organs of the human body, the skin is not a uniform tissue; rather, it is composed of cellular layers of different kinds which lie one under the other.

Essentially, the skin is divided into three layers: the epidermis, the corium, and the hypodermis. Most cosmetic preparations come into contact only with the outermost layer of the epidermis, called the *stratum corneum*.

This layer consists of "horny" cells which are flat and colorless. They are almost parallel to the skin surface and are arranged in layers much like tiles in a roof. These cells have no nucleus, a very low moisture content, and are dead in the sense that no metabolic processes occur in them. They are constantly being shed, and contain an epidermic fatty material which renders them supple and waterproof.

The next two layers of the epidermis are the *stratum lucidum* and the *stratum granulosum*. Between them lies a thin, continuous membrane called Rein's barrier, which acts as a definite demarcation between the corneal layers and the deeper-lying skin tissues.

Penetrating the barrier is a must for ingredients such as vitamins and hormones which are intended to act in depth. Some substances will effect this penetration; others will not. It would do no good to spread a hormone cream on the surface of the skin if that cream were unable to penetrate to the depth where it could do its work. The dead layers certainly would not make use of it.

Determining what ingredients will penetrate and produce desired results has consumed monumental time on the part of many researchers. To send active ingredients to the depth where they can be effective, cosmetic chemists add them to a base material which can handle the problem of penetration.

The next questions are the important ones. Do the active ingredients really make a difference in the condition of the skin? Will we look more youthful for using them?

Not very many years ago one read that there was no substantial evidence that vitamins or hormones added to a cosmetic were effective in treating the skin. One may still read this. There have been two opposing points of view on the subject. One holds that cosmetics with depth effect are really over-rated; that hormones could have unfortunate side effects so should be used with utmost care; and, finally that no cosmetic preparation is going to restore youth. On the other hand, the view is equally one-sided: every new active ingredient reported to be effective should be welcomed with absolute joy and confidence; those who doubt are only unhappy because they didn't discover it first.

Somewhere in between, responsible cosmetic chemists attempt to determine just how effective these important active ingredients are when it comes to working in depth. The field is one of the newest and most exciting in cosmetics, and one to follow with great interest.

So much for the debate. What about the answer? Are you wasting money on preparations with vitamins, hormones, or other active ingredients?

Probably not. Evidence now suggests that there is definite beneficial effect from the use of certain hormones and vitamins in cosmetic preparations. The evidence has been a long time coming, and exact determination of the kind and extent of effects provides continued controversy and research opportunities.

Biopsies have indicated that external application of estrogens increases skin thickness, enhances texture, color, and blood supply.

Evaluation of such preparations is a complex matter. Biologically active materials that are effective underneath the surface of the skin produce what cosmetic chemists call "observable results" only after some time. It is much simpler to judge whether or not a hand-softener really works than whether or not a hormone cream takes years off a woman's looks.

The effect of hormones on the skin has long been known, for hormone changes at puberty provoke observable changes in the skin of teen-agers, and menstrual changes in older women are every bit as telling in the appearance of the skin. Experiments continue with sex hormones for cosmetic application.

In studying cosmetic use of vitamins, the effect of oral application comes into play. Vitamin deficiency in the body is often apparent in changes in the skin; however, this does not *necessarily* mean that topical applications (external use) of vitamins will be effective in restoring the skin to a healthy condition. When vitamin deficiency occurs, the whole body must be treated. Where the skin itself is the problem (open sores, cuts, rashes, etc.), topical application of an ointment containing vitamins can be effective in promoting healing.

Some vitamins are considered to be effective by some researchers and are being used today in quality products. Other vitamins, thus far judged valueless for cosmetic use, are passed over by those who formulate cosmetics.

Vitamins and hormones are not the only deep effect ingredients being studied. Others include enzymes, proteins, peptones, peptides, and amino acids. And there are more.

How is a consumer to judge the new preparations with such fantastic, wonder-making claims made for them? Probably she can't. Cosmetic chemists themselves do not agree on the value of many ingredients and preparations. Still, the consumer now knows that certain deep-acting ingredients can effect beneficial changes. She knows also that manufacturers subject their preparations to extensive testing before putting them on the market. She can assume, therefore, that these marvelous new products are probably safe to use, and that some are worth giving a try (if the advertising claims make reasonable sense and if the cost is not prohibitive).

Something else to think about in this search for youth is that conscientious care with old standbys plus use of, perhaps, a wrinkle-fighting, lanolin-rich lubricating cream, can work wonders. Regular care is, after all and before all, the answer to a healthier, younger-looking skin. Sporadic splurges with expensive, highly touted miracle creams probably won't serve as well in the long run.

9

Preparations to Beautify

If the skillful application of makeup couldn't transform Plain Jane into Glamorous Greta, a lot of talented Hollywood and New York makeup artists would be seeking new ways of becoming rich. But the fact of the matter is that makeup *can* effect such transformations.

And, while most women cannot afford to visit exclusive salons for an expensive makeup job each time they want to play bridge with the girls, most can afford a simple lesson in the art of makeup from a skilled cosmetician.

The secret to making the most of your looks is in understanding your own face and features, and in learning how best to use makeup to enhance good and minimize bad points. Learning such things as whether your face looks better with a natural brow line or a slightly altered one will make a big difference in your appearance. Is your natural lip line becoming, or should you accent too-thin lips by "painting on" a wider mouth? Is your face an oval, square, round, or elongated shape? Are your eyes well spaced? Nose too long? Cheekbones too prominent?

Although it is possible to analyze your own bone structure and facial features, a more objective viewpoint is best—if you can afford that one lesson from a cosmetician. For those who want to experiment with makeup techniques on their own, a few minutes spent with charts showing how to treat specific problems will be well spent. Shading tricks can turn a square face into a more pleasing oval. Charts show just how and where to apply shading to create this effect. How best to arch brows and to shadow eyes can be learned in the same way.

There are those who object to any alteration of natural lines, for one reason or another. But one might well ask in return just why makeup should be used at all if not to create the most pleasing effects.

Not that one should paint on an entirely new face. There is a considerable difference between using makeup to enhance certain features and in trying to design an entirely new look that nature never intended. Imagine how demoralizing it would be at the end of the day to cream off makeup and peel off false eyelashes and discover that, underneath it all, there was the same old you. The transition from stranger to self would be devastating, especially if one faced it each day.

Remember that makeup should be a suggestion, not

an out-and-out statement. It must be subtle. Even with eye makeup, which demands a more dramatic touch than other kinds of makeup, one should avoid harsh, definitive lines. This is all part of the art of makeup—achieving a look that is truly lovely through subtle and skillful use of available materials and techniques.

Something else to keep in mind is that cosmetics go in and out of fashion in much the same way as wardrobes. One year eyeliner is in vogue and the next it is out. White lipstick, deep purple, brown, or bright red may be the thing this year and taboo next.

While women enjoy being in style cosmetically, they must always take into consideration their own facial—and life—styles. A *Vogue* model may be smashing indeed with shaved brows and purple and red eye shadow, but for the mother of three in Sioux Falls, the look is something less than appropriate.

The challenge in all of this lies in learning how to beautify through makeup preparations without looking artificial or like someone other than yourself. Lynda Bird Johnson was still as much Miss Johnson after her famed visit to George Masters' salon as she was before—she was just a lot more glamorous. Syndicated columnist Erma Bombeck, who writes of everyday life among the hausfrau set, tells of eating an abundance of spaghetti and still not looking like gorgeous Sophia Loren. Most of us could paint those magnificently arched brows on our faces and use eyeliner to sketch almond-shaped eyes and still not look like Sophia, spaghetti or no. We must learn to be our best-looking selves and not an imitation of anyone else.

Just what is makeup? The term comes from the history of the theater, where features had to be exaggerated in order for the audience to perceive anything at all of the facial expressions of the performers. In other days and in other times, makeup has been called by different terms, but throughout history and by whatever name, it has been associated with the theater.

Until the mid-1920's the popular notion that cosmetics were at best immoral meant that only a tinted, lightly scented face powder was acceptable to America's "polite" society. But with the advent of the early film stars and a new look at glamour, makeup lost much of its unfortunate image. Along with powder, women were able to wear rouge and lipstick without being considered "floozies."

Without counting, try a quick estimate of the number of cosmetic preparations the average woman uses regularly. A good guess would be around two dozen. Most women, use, regularly, at least two kinds of creams, a mask, a toning lotion or astringent, a foundation cream or makeup base (or both), powder, a blush or rouge, eyeliner, eye shadow, eyelash mascara, and brow mascara. They also use bath oils or foams, perfumes, nail lacquers and remover, hand lotions, cuticle removers, shampoos, hair conditioners and rinses, dipilatories or shaving creams, anti-perspirants and several deodorants. Many also use a number of expensive creams they hope will take years off their face and make wrinkles disappear.

The woman who spends considerable time using these preparations and a portion of her budget buying them, should learn as much about them as possible—about their formulations and what they are supposed to accomplish.

Here are some of the basics found in most cosmetic cabinets: face makeup, eye makeup, nail preparations, and fragrances.

FACE MAKEUP

FOUNDATION MAKEUPS are precisely that—foundations that conceal imperfections, protect the skin, and provide a base for application of finishing touches. They generally have a color that is slightly darker than the skin color and a creamy consistency that leaves the skin feeling soft and comfortable.

Major ingredients are oils, waxes, titanium dioxide, kaolin, and pigment colors.

Skin color changes from one time of the year to another. The wise woman takes these changes into account when using (and making) cosmetics and changes her foundation from time to time. Foundation makeup must blend well and must look natural in order for the total look to be becoming.

FACE POWDERS are used over a foundation to achieve a smooth, matte finish. Many a peaches and cream complexion looks delicious because of this important finishing touch. To be effective, face powder must be light and silky, spreading easily and clinging to the skin.

The major ingredient of most face powders is talc. Other ingredients vary according to the manufacturer. Zinc stearate is added to increase bulk, aid adhesion, and resist moisture; also added are titanium dioxide, a white pigment that helps hide imperfections, and other pigments to create the desired powder shades. Small amounts of almond or other oil help adhesion and stabilize color. The fine texture desired in face powders comes from the mixing process.

Most popular in contemporary cosmetics is a light, fluffy powder that gives a translucent effect. Other powder styles include the heavier, the more opaque, and the lustrous or glistening powders.

ROUGE is used to give a natural looking blush to the cheeks. A chemical binder holds pigments, talc, and other ingredients for "dry" or compact rouge. A cream, or paste rouge has pigments ground with oil and waxes to form a smooth consistency. Until recently, rouge was made in quite a variety of colors; however, one frequently finds a single "blush" rouge in a line of cosmetics, designed to suit all complexions.

It takes some experimenting with rouge, as it does with face powder, to achieve exactly the desired look. A shortcut to manufacturing either rouge or powder is to have a sample of a shade you like best, then work toward matching it with your own product.

LIPSTICKS are creamy sticks made of waxes, fats, oils, and pigments. They may have special formulations to soften and protect or to achieve some other desired effect. They are made by grinding the pigments and combining them with melted waxes and oils. The heated product is poured into a mold where it hardens to a state that allows it to resist breaking and melting.

Pigments used in lipsticks are skin-staining dyes that are non-toxic and certified safe for cosmetic use. Helping the color stay on the lips and supplying viscosity is castor oil. Other ingredients give the product desired sheen and consistency.

EYE MAKEUP

Eye makeup is becoming more and more important each year, for women are fast learning that emphasizing the eyes is the most effective beauty trick in 5000 years. Although Cleopatra used eye cosmetics unsparingly, that kind of use has been out of style for centuries, returning only recently. Today, fashion magazines are full of photographs of beautiful women disguised behind green and purple eyelids (sometimes with the paint extending to the temples and decorated with pasted on sequins and jewels), or with countenances altered by oriental eyes in a Caucasian setting.

It isn't necessary to try to rival the Queen of the Nile or anybody else in the amount of eye makeup used, but it is necessary to have a variety of colors and kinds of eye makeup available to achieve the look you have in mind.

EYE SHADOW is a cream or cake cosmetic applied to the lids (and sometimes to the area under the eye) to emphasize the eyes. It can be made in any color, and is frequently sold in "ensembles" where a trio of shades of the same color is packaged together. Popular shades are grays, blues, browns, greens, and smoky grayish-purples.

Shadows are usually made of lanolin, spermaceti, and petrolatum combined with colors. Pearl-like effects are created by adding one of the most unlikely sounding of all cosmetic ingredients—fish scale essence.

MASCARA is used to darken lashes and eyebrows. It has the same purpose as shadow—to accent the eyes and to make the whites look brighter.

Mascara usually consists of a mixture of color, fats, waxes, and emulsifying agents. Cake mascara is applied with a wet brush. Cream or liquid mascaras are similar, but are made to suit the kind of application desired.

EYEBROW PENCILS AND LINERS are primarily a combination of colors and waxes made into sticks or encased in special containers. Liners can be in liquid or cake form as well. Both pencils as well as other forms of liners must be relatively waterproof.

EYE MAKEUP REMOVER can be made of a combination of ingredients or a single ingredient. Its purpose is simply to remove makeup efficiently and safely from the eye area. Since the eye must be protected from irritating substances, safety should be the primary criterion in selecting a cleanser.

NAIL PREPARATIONS

Nail preparations are as much a part of the cosmetic scene as are powder and mascara. Early manicures consisted of few nail preparations and an abundance of effort. Nails were filed to an oval shape, then buffed with a chamois-covered buffer and a polishing powder of stannic oxide with chalk and a little jeweler's rouge.

For women today who face a constant battle with brittle, splitting, or layering nails, the old-style manicure is still one of the best approaches to problem nails. Chamois-covered buffers are back in style and are available at beauty shops around the country.

NAIL LACQUERS are composed chiefly of nitrocellulose, which is made flexible by the addition of plasticizers. Natural and synthetic resins make modern nail lacquers more durable and lustrous; gums make them adherent. As is true with lipsticks, nail lacquer colors go in and out of style with the seasons.

We hesitate to suggest home manufacture of nail lacquer because of the risks of grinding and dispersing nitrocellulose and because of certain solvent hazards. In fact, many manufacturers of cosmetics have their nail varnish compounded for them by outside lacquer firms whose business it is to deal with these problems.

The nails are lifeless, in the same sense as is hair. There is neither circulation in the nails nor are there nerves. Strong alkaline solutions and prolonged contact with detergent solutions are said to make them brittle, and most women will agree with this observation. Keeping lovely nails is a problem for a great many women. As is true with other beauty routines, regular care is part of the answer to nail problems.

NAIL POLISH REMOVERS are unique among cosmetic cleaners. Whereas skin and hair cleaners must tackle a variety of kinds of soil, nail cleaners must remove only lacquers.

Solvents especially designed for this chore clean the surface of the nail and avoid leaving it sticky or brittle. Most lacquers have fat added to combat a strong drying effect. Typical are lanolin, fatty alcohols, and vegetable oils.

Since lacquer removers are volatile, they should be used with care and should be kept tightly capped while not in use to prevent evaporation.

FRAGRANCES

Volumes have been written about the special aura that is woman, about the sweetly scented bodies that drive men to distraction. There is no denying the impact of a personal fragrance that whispers something special about the wearer. It invites remembering. It says something distinctive. And it is totally feminine.

Even if your goal is not driving men to distraction (perhaps it is just to the train station), using perfume or cologne regularly accomplishes something special. It makes a woman feel like a woman. It makes a man know she is a woman. And what, after all, is more to the point when it comes to using cosmetics?

Perfumery is an art. Can you practice it at home? Of course you can, but if you choose to do it in the style of the professionals, it will require a substantial investment. You can also choose to do it as an amateur, a method almost cost-free and perhaps as exciting.

Formulas included here represent both kinds of perfume-making, the amateur and the professional. There is the technique for truly creative perfumery, a formula for a versatile cream cologne, and the formula reported to be a twin of that for Jean Patou's "Joy."

Here is a brief overview of the elements of the art and the processes involved in perfumery:

NATURAL PERFUMES are the products of plant metabolism. In its highest form, natural perfume is found in the scent of fresh flowers, but it is also found in leaves, stems, barks, wood, roots, rhizomes, fruits, seeds, gums, etc. The odoriferous part of the plant generally occurs as a volatile oil, which, after processing, becomes a highly aromatic liquid.

ISOLATES are the extracted natural products.

SYNTHETICS are built up from other substances, chemically synthesized to produce a scent like the natural one. An example is ionone, which has the odor of violets and which is synthesized from citral and acetone.

ARTIFICIAL FLOWER OILS are blends of natural flower extracts, synthetics, balsams, and animal extracts. They are widely used in perfumery, not only for finished perfumes but also for scenting cosmetics.

FINISHED PERFUMES are prepared from the artificial flower oils in a solution of about 80 percent alcohol. They are blended with balsams, gums, certain resins, and animal extracts. Additional flower extracts may be added to enhance the finished product. Perfumes are "aged" in tanks until they mature.

Processes for collecting the natural oils include distillation, expression, and, most familiar, extraction, which includes maceration and enfleurage.

For the amateur who wants to try truly creative perfumery, that is, starting from the flower petals, enfleurage is the process to use. A form of enfleurage is still used in some French perfume factories.

FACE MAKEUP

Foundation Cream

This foundation cream has a beautiful, non-greasy texture. It is an excellent powder base that allows a smooth, even covering of powder to cling to the skin.

Lanolin	*1 teaspoon*
Stearic acid	*1 tablespoon plus 2 1/2 teaspoons*
Triethanolamine	*1/4 teaspoon*
Distilled water	*1/4 cup*
Diethylene glycol monoethyl ether	*2 teaspoons*

Heat lanolin and stearic acid in top of double boiler to a temperature of 185°F (85°C). Heat triethanolamine, water, and diethylene glycol monoethyl ether in another double boiler to the same temperature, then add to lanolin mixture, while stirring. Remove from heat and continue stirring until cream reaches 77–86°F (25–30°C), and package. Since this cream is used as a foundation, and since perfumed products (makeup base and/or powder) usually will be applied, it is suggested that this cream not be perfumed. However, if perfume is desired, add it prior to packaging. *Yield: 1/2 cup.*

Pigmented Foundation Cream

This foundation cream works as do other foundations: it creates a protective and uniform base for the application of makeup or powder. The added advantage of a pigmented foundation cream is that it has light covering powder, concealing minor blemishes and imperfections in the skin. Used below the eyes, it is effective in hiding dark circles.

Mineral oil	*1 tablespoon*
Beeswax	*1/2 teaspoon*
Ceresine wax	*1/4 teaspoon*
Arlacel 186	*3/4 teaspoon*
Sorbo	*2 tablespoons*
Titanium dioxide	*1 teaspoon*
Distilled water	*2 tablespoons plus 1 teaspoon*

Heat mineral oil, beeswax, ceresine wax, Arlacel 186, and Sorbo in the top of a double boiler to a temperature of 158°F (70°C). Blend in the titanium dioxide until it is uniformly dispersed. Heat water to a temperature of 162°F (72°C), then add to other ingredients, blending until cool. You may "homogenize" by using an egg beater to increase the smoothness. *Yield: 1/2 cup.*

Cream Makeup

This makeup allows you to work with the tint to adjust it to the color that is just right for you. The cream is made first, then put on your glass plate where you add titanium dioxide (the covering agent) and kaolin. After these are worked into the cream with a stiff spatula, pigment is added. You will want to use the flesh tones and should experiment with a tiny pinch at a time. As you work the pigments into the cream, you can easily reach the shade you wish.

Something to remember is this—commercially made makeups are milled; yours are made with glass plate and metal spatula, so they are not going to be as smooth in application as the preparations you buy. You must be careful to apply them evenly, working them onto the skin and blending smoothly.

Mineral oil	*1 3/4 teaspoons*
Beeswax	*3/4 teaspoon*
Synthetic spermaceti wax	*1/2 teaspoon*
Ceresine wax	*1/2 teaspoon*
Lanolin	*3/4 teaspoon*
Borax	*1/5 of 1/4 teaspoon*
Distilled water	*1 tablespoon plus 1/2 teaspoon*
Titanium dioxide	*1/3 of 1/4 teaspoon*
Kaolin	*1/4 teaspoon*
Pigment, as desired	

Heat mineral oil, beeswax, spermaceti wax, ceresine wax, and lanolin in top of double boiler to a temperature of 167°F (75°C), or until all waxes are melted. Dissolve borax in water and heat to a temperature of 158°F (70°C), then add to oil and wax mixture and stir slowly until temperature drops to 86°F (30°C). Perfume lightly if you wish, remembering that perfumed powder will probably be worn with this makeup.

Pour cream onto glass plate. Work titanium dioxide and kaolin into the cream base with a spatula. Add pigment and work well until the desired shade is reached. Working in the pigment and getting a smooth, lovely cream takes time and effort, but the finished product is well worth it. *Yield: 1/8 cup.*

Liquid Makeup

Liquid makeup is probably one of the most popular cosmetics on the market. It is easy to apply and makes a good base for face powders.

This formula requires some experimentation, for the pigments are added to the makeup while it is cooking. Unlike the cream makeup, which allows you to adjust the tint to a desired color, this one requires that you come up with the right tint on the first guess since once the pigments are added, you have your final color. Some experimenting with pigments will give you the color you want— it just takes a bit of experience.

Sodium lauryl *sulfate*	*1/4 teaspoon*
Bentonite	*1/4 teaspoon*
Kaoline	*1/2 teaspoon*
Pigments	*1 teaspoon*

Mineral oil	*1 tablespoon plus 1/2 teaspoon*
Propylene glycol monostearate	*1 1/4 teaspoons*
Stearic acid	*1/2 teaspoon*
Triethanolamine	*1/4 teaspoon*
Distilled water	*3 tablespoons plus 1 1/2 teaspoons*

Grind in mortar (or work on glass plate with stiff spatula) the sodium lauryl sulfate, bentonite, kaolin, and pigments. Put aside.

Melt in top of double boiler the mineral oil, propylene glycol monostearate, and stearic acid to a temperature of 167°F (75°C). In a second double boiler, heat triethanolamine and water to the same temperature. Add the mineral oil mixture to the water solution, while stirring. When the emulsion has cooled to 130°F (55°C), stir in the pulverized mixture of sodium lauryl sulfate, bentonite, kaolin, and pigments. Add perfume, if desired, at 113°F (45°C), and stir. Transfer to mortar, and grind to room temperature. Let stand a day or two before using. *Yield: 1/3 cup.*

Face Powders

Can fine face powders be made at home? Absolutely! Face powders are among the most satisfactory homemade cosmetics—fun to make, delightful to use. They require mixing with mortar and pestle in order to achieve a pleasing consistency. Homemade powders are almost as silky as those that are commercially made. They can be exactly the color you wish and carry the scent that is distinctively yours.

Three formulas are given: a light, translucent face powder (probably the most popular of today's powders), a medium powder, and a powder with matte finish that covers minor skin imperfections.

FACE POWDER, TRANSLUCENT

Talc	*4 tablespoons*
Zinc oxide	*1/2 teaspoon*
Zinc stearate	*2 teaspoons*
Precipitated chalk	*2 teaspoons*
Pigments, as desired	
Perfume, as desired	

Put all ingredients except color and perfume into a mortar. Rub down well, then add pigments. Keep working until color is desired shade, then add perfume by drops and keep working until powder is of desired consistency. *Yield: 1/3 cup.*

FACE POWDER, MEDIUM

Precipitated chalk	*1/2 teaspoon*
Titanium dioxide	*1/2 teaspoon*
Talc	*3 tablespoons*
Zinc stearate	*2 teaspoons*
Almond oil	*2 teaspoons*
Pigments, as desired	
Perfume, as desired	

Follow directions for translucent powder. *Yield: 1/4 cup.*

FACE POWDER, MATTE

Talc	*4 tablespoons*
Zinc oxide	*2 teaspoons*

Zinc stearate	*2 teaspoons*
Precipitated chalk	*2 tablespoons*
Pigments, as desired	
Perfume, as desired	

Follow directions for translucent powder. *Yield: 1/2 cup.*

Blush Rouge

This a beautiful preparation, both in application and in appearance. This is one time you should go against the "pinch at a time" method of coloring, for in order to get the blush look popular today, the cream needs to appear a deep red in the jar. On the face, it becomes a lovely, natural blush. We recommend beginning with about 3/4 teaspoon of pigment. After the mixture is removed from the heat and is cooled, try on the face to test the color. If it isn't dark enough, then simply remelt the mixture in a double boiler and add more pigment. This is an extremely simple preparation to make and is almost foolproof because color can be easily adjusted to desired richness.

Beeswax	*1/2 teaspoon*
Stearic acid	*3/4 teaspoon*
Cetyl alcohol	*1/2 teaspoon*
Petrolatum	*3 tablespoons*
Mineral oil	*3/4 teaspoon*
Pigment, as desired (we like a D & C Red #6, barium lake)	

Melt all ingredients together in top of double boiler. Stir until color is uniform and mixture is smooth. See comments above about adjusting color to suit.   *Yield: 1/4 cup.*

Lipstick

This is the most complicated (but not difficult) formula to make in the kitchen. Step-by-step instructions are offered for making a smooth, creamy lipstick that feels good on the lips and that rivals quality lipsticks on today's cosmetics counter.

Experimenting with lipstick colors is great fun. Try matching a lipstick to a special costume or try inventing a brand new color. Anything is possible.

Don't undertake this project at 9 P.M. after a busy day. Plan to work on lipstick when there is ample time to enjoy the project.

This lipstick can be either a "paint pot" lipstick poured into small jars or a stick lipstick. The formula makes enough so that you can pour a stick *and* have a small paint pot if you choose.

A word to the wise. *Go lightly with pigments;* a pinch or two goes a long way. You can always add a bit more color, but once it is in the mixture, it is too late to decide there is too much color. If, for instance, you want a pale coral, you'll be starting with an orange pigment. Use a pinch, then work from there. You may wish to blend several pigments to get exactly the shade you want. In this case, blend the dry pigments on a corner of your glass plate until you think you have about the shade you want.

There are two parts to this lipstick, the absorption base and the lipstick base. The absorption base is made first, then the lipstick base.

ABSORPTION BASE

Span 80	*2 teaspoons*
Ceresine wax	*3 1/4 teaspoons*
Petrolatum	*1 tablespoon plus 2 teaspoons*
Mineral oil	*3 tablespoons plus 1 1/2 teaspoons*
Lanolin	*2 1/4 teaspoons*

Put all ingredients into the top of a double boiler and heat until melted. Sir until the mixture reaches 149°F (65°C). Set aside to cool.

LIPSTICK BASE

Beeswax	*1/2 teaspoon*
Synthetic spermaceti wax	*1/8 teaspoon*
Ceresine wax	*1 teaspoon*
Carnauba wax	*1/4 teaspoon*
Mineral oil	*1/2 teaspoon*
Castor oil	*1 1/2 teaspoons*
Absorption base (above)	*1 teaspoon*
Pigments, as desired	

Heat beeswax, spermaceti wax, ceresine wax, carnauba wax, mineral oil, and castor oil in top of double boiler until melted. Let stand until cool and solid, preferably for at least an hour. Then remelt and add 1 teaspoon of the absorption base, stirring well. Let stand again until cool.

Put pigments on a corner of a glass plate. Remember, just a pinch will probably do the trick if you are looking for a pale color. The new bright reds will, of course, require more. Add a drop or two of additional castor oil to the pigments and work into a runny paste. Put a small amount of lipstick base mixture (the second mixture) on the plate. Using a stiff metal spatula, spread the base out on the glass plate and work until smooth. Smear it out and then pick it up again, in long, even strokes. When the base is smooth, work in enough pigments to give the desired shade. Your lipstick must be smooth.

Work in more of the absorption base until the proper texture is reached, until it has the desired creaminess. When the lipstick has a good sheen and seems entirely smooth, it is ready. Put it back into the top of the double boiler and heat until melted. Remove from heat and stir well. Perfume slightly (if you choose) and pour into desired container. Use small jars or old lipstick tubes, cleaned and turned until the circular "platform" that holds the lipstick is at the bottom of the tube. You will want to shape the end of the stick over a flame or with a knife, working carefully. Use a brush to apply paint pot lipstick. *Yield: 2–3 tubes.*

EYE MAKEUP

Cream Eye Shadow

This creamy smooth eye shadow is marvelous. Its texture is pleasing (not too stiff and not too soft) and its color possibilities almost unlimited. It may be applied with a brush or with your finger. Use only *inorganic cosmetic colorants* in this and in all eye preparations. (See discussion on colorants in "Perfumes, Colors, and Preservatives," p. 36.)

BASE

Lanolin	*1 teaspoon*
Synthetic spermaceti wax	*1 1/4 teaspoons*
Petrolatum	*2 tablespoons plus 1 1/2 teaspoons*

Melt lanolin, spermaceti, and petrolatum in the top of a double boiler.

COLOR

Pigment	*1/4 teaspoon at a time until desired color is reached*
Zinc oxide	*1/2 teaspoon*
Base (*above*)	*sufficient*

Blend pigment with zinc oxide (white) until desired color is reached. Add to base while still warm.

Place cooled mass on glass plate and work well with stiff spatula. Work until grainy texture and streaks are removed. You may, if desired, add more pigment or more zinc oxide to the shadow while working on the glass plate, but try to keep additions at this point to a minimum. When you have worked shadow to smooth, uniformly colored cream, put into a small container. It will become firmer in a day or two.

Suggested colors: brown, beige, tan, blue, green bronze, silver. To obtain scintillating effects, add small amounts of powdered gold leaf, bronze powder, aluminum powder, or fish scale essence. *Yield: 1/8 cup.*

Powder Eye Shadow

This great shadow may be packaged as a loose powder or as a dry cake. Color possibilities include the browns, grays, greens, blues, and metallics. Only *inorganic cos-*

metic colorants may be used. (See "Perfumes, Colors, and Preservatives" for information on eye colorants, p. 36.)

Talc	*1 tablespoon plus 2 teaspoons*
Titanium dioxide	*1/4 teaspoon*
Zinc stearate	*1 1/2 teaspoons*
Kaolin	*3/4 teaspoon*
Pigment	*up to 1 1/2 teaspoons*

Place ingredients, except pigments, in mortar and rub down well. Add pigment a little at a time, working well each time until desired shade is obtained.   *Yield: 1/8 cup.*

Cake Mascara No. 1

Two cake mascaras with very different ingredients are given below. Both are quite satisfactory products, and both pour into smooth, solid cakes. This first formula is somewhat easier to prepare, although neither is difficult. Mascara should be applied with a wet brush and will dry on the lashes.

Only *inorganic cosmetic colorants* can be used safely in eye preparations. (See the notes on eye colorants in "Perfumes, Colors, and Preservatives," p. 36.)

Stearic acid	*1 1/2 teaspoons*
Triethanolamine	*1/8 teaspoon*
Beeswax	*1 3/4 teaspoons*
Carnauba wax	*2 3/4 teaspoons*
Pigment (cosmetic black or other)	*1 teaspoon*

Put all ingredients in the top of a double boiler and melt, stirring well. Pour into mold. Molds may be formed by pressing aluminum foil in the bottom of a muffin tin. When mixture cools and hardens, remove the foil and you will have a nice, solid cake. Allow to cool slowly. Cake should not be more than 1/4-inch thick. *Yield: 1/8 cup.*

Cake Mascara No. 2

In making this smooth mascara, do not worry when tiny soap bubbles begin rising—they are supposed to do just that. Earlier mascaras sometimes used soaps as emulsifiers, and these caused eye irritation. Both formulas given here should not cause any irritation to those who use them, so there should be no concern about having "soap" near the eyes.

Do take care in the stirring process to avoid concentration of pigment. Please see the note above on using inorganic cosmetic colorants for cake mascaras.

Stearic acid	*2 tablespoons plus 1/2 teaspoon*
Pigment (cosmetic black or other)	*1/4 teaspoon*
Triethanolamine	*2 3/4 teaspoons*
Arlacel 165	*scant 1/2 teaspoon*
Castor oil	*1/8 teaspoon*

Melt stearic acid and color in top of double boiler to a temperature of 167°F (75°C). Heat triethanolamine over water to the same temperature, then add to stearic acid in a thin stream, stirring until tiny soap bubbles begin to rise. Add Arlacel 165 and castor oil and stir until thoroughly mixed. Remove from heat and continue stirring. Be sure pigment is not concentrated in center of mixture. Pour into mold while still warm. (See remarks above on making molds.) *Yield: 1/4 cup.*

Mascara Crayon

This crayon may be used as an eyeliner. It draws a good, even line without crumbling or caking. The problem with this homemade preparation is packaging. We have come up with an idea we like: use two sipping straws (preferably stiff paper) to make a crayon holder. Perhaps you can discover an even better method.

Paraffin wax	*1 tablespoon*
Carnauba wax	*1/2 teaspoon*
Beeswax	*2 teaspoons*
Petrolatum	*1 1/2 teaspoons*
Lanolin	*1 teaspoon*
Cetyl alcohol (1-hexadecanol)	*1 teaspoon*
Pigment, as desired *	*3/4 teaspoon*

Place all ingredients in top of double boiler, place over heat, and melt. Stir to ensure complete dispersion of pigment. When temperature reaches 158–167°F (70–75°C), remove from heat.

Make a slit the full length of one straw, then slip it

---

* Only *inorganic cosmetic colorants* may be used. (See "Perfumes, Colors, and Preservatives" for information on colorants for eye preparations, p. 36.)

inside the second straw. Place a paper clip at one end to seal it closed. Stand straws upright in a paper cup (the cup will catch spills).

Carefully remove melted mixture from the heat and pour slowly (it will pour in a steady, thin stream) into straws. When cooled, remove the outer straw. Peel the inner straw (working from the slit) away from the end of the crayon, and, with razor blade or sharp knife, cut the end at an angle to make a good drawing edge. *Yield: 1/4 cup.*

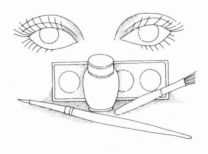

Eye Makeup Remover

For obvious reasons, most eye makeup is not water soluble. This means that eye makeup remover must have a solvency that will cleanse the materials used in this particular kind of makeup. A harsh solvent would be entirely inappropriate for this delicate chore. An ideal material is a low viscosity, fully refined white mineral oil. Using a fresh cotton pad or ball moistened with the oil, wipe away eye makeup.

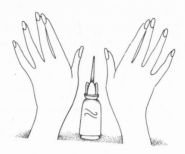

NAIL PREPARATIONS

Nail Buffing Paste

Buffing pastes are truly old-fashioned cosmetics. They are among the most effective nail beauty treatments, helping to keep nails strong and pretty, and guarding against splitting, layering, and breaking.

ABRASIVE POLISH

Stannic oxide	*2 tablespoons*
Powdered silica	*2 teaspoons*
Butyl stearate or oleic acid	*1 teaspoon*

PASTE

Gum tragacanth	*1/4 teaspoon*
Glycerin	*2 tablespoons*
Color, as desired	
Perfume, as desired	

Mix stannic oxide, powdered silica, and butyl stearate (or oleic acid) in mortar. Rub down well and put aside. Mix the gum tragacanth and glycerin thoroughly in a glass, then let stand for 1 to 2 hours. It will thicken to a gummy mucilage.

Empty abrasive powders from mortar onto glass plate. Add mucilage, and, with stiff spatula, work into powders, using enough mucilage to achieve desired consistency.

Finally, add a touch of color and a drop or two of perfume (if desired) and work into the mixture. When color is evenly dispersed, package in small container. *Yield: 1/3 cup.*

Nail Polish Remover

This cleanser for the nails consists of substances that dissolve nail lacquer, the job which all polish removers must accomplish without harming the surface of the nails and without leaving the surface dry and brittle. This is an efficient, satisfactory cleanser for a specific grooming step.

Ethyleneglycol monoethyl ether	*1/4 cup*
Butyl acetate	*2 tablespoons*
Propylene glycol	*1 teaspoon*
Castor oil	*1 teaspoon*

Stir together until well blended, then bottle. *Yield: 1/2 cup.*

FRAGRANCES

Homemade Perfumes

You can try making your own perfumes at home by the enfleurage method. Instructions are simple and go back hundreds of years.

Place a thin covering of pure lard on your glass plate, then cover with lightly placed flower petals. Store in a dark place for about 24 hours, then remove and discard flowers. Replace them with fresh flowers. Repeat the process for several days, then heat the lard just enough to melt it and mix it with a like amount of ethyl alcohol. Pour into bottle and be certain cap is tightly closed. Store for two to three weeks, then pour off the scented alcohol, which is your do-it-yourself perfume. The fat left behind is called a pomade.

What you don't have in *your* perfume are those ingredients mentioned above that tone and give persistence to perfumes. But, since you are not planning to store it for ages or to put it on the market, this is of small concern.

Cream Cologne

Here is a chance to experiment with perfumes. The cream base can be scented with any perfume or combination of perfumes to achieve a fragrance that is totally you. Begin with a teaspoon of perfume, then add more until you are satisfied with the fragrance level. If you are making it for a gift (and it does make an ideal gift) prepare it a couple of weeks in advance of gift day so that the fragrance has an opportunity to mellow.

Glyceryl monostearate	*3/4 teaspoon*
Stearic acid	*1/2 teaspoon*
Mineral oil	*1 tablespoon plus 1/2 teaspoon*
Triethanolamine	*1/4 teaspoon*
Distilled water	*3/4 cup*
Perfume, *as desired*	

Heat glyceryl monostearate, stearic acid, and mineral oil in top of double boiler to a temperature of 158°F (70°C). Solids should be melted. In another pan, heat triethanolamine and water to the same temperature; then add to first mixture, while stirring. Stir until entire mixture reaches a temperature of 113°F (45°C). Perfume and pour into suitable container. *Yield: 1 cup.*

"Pure Joy"

Cost is a major consideration if you are serious about trying real perfume-making. If you can find several people to share your hobby, then you can purchase the relatively expensive ingredients at reasonable cost. The cost of the finished perfume is anything but extravagant—the problem lies in having to buy large amounts of individual ingredients.

In a story released July 7, 1971, by the Los Angeles Times News Service, it was reported that a woman's liberation group at Columbia University was making "Pure Joy," a perfume called a twin of Jean Patou's famed "Joy," one of the world's most expensive perfumes. The cost of making "Pure Joy" is $3 an ounce; cost of buying "Joy" is about $65 an ounce.

Here's the formula, as it was revealed to the public:

Heliotropin	*1/2 dram*
Oil of rose	*2 1/2 drams*
Synthetic bergamot oil	*1 dram*
Musk	*4 drops*
Ambergris	*2/10 dram*
Artificial jasmine	*2/10 dram*
Neroli oil	*4 drops*
Angelica	*8 drops*
Vetivert	*8 drops*
Medium perfume oil base	*3 ounces*

Blend all ingredients.   *Yield: approximately 3 1/2 ounces.*

10

Preparations for Grooming

Bush-country women who rub rancid fats into their hair to make it "clean" and lovely, and elegant San Franciscans who spend small fortunes in exclusive beauty salons are all after the same thing—they just go about it differently and with different degrees of sophistication. The object is to be attractive and desirable. And, while most of the folks we know wouldn't think much of the fat-in-the-hair technique, it pleases those who use it and their admirers.

To be attractive and desirable, a woman begins by grooming, or preparing her body. For most people, this means beginning with cleanliness, which, whether or not it is next to godliness, is certainly next to prettiness.

Our healthy bodies take an active interest in being

clean. Surface impurities are disposed of by the constant sloughing off of the uppermost "horny" cells of the skin, and impurities that are below the surface make their way there in order that they may be disposed of in the same fashion. Hair is cleansed, in a sense, by continuous self-renewal, with old hair shed and replaced by new. In the mouth, saliva has a certain cleansing effect on the teeth, and bacterial matter assists in the decomposition of food particles left there.

But of course all of this is not enough. The most unpopular person in any crowd is the fellow who has relied on nature alone to keep him fresh and lovely.

Grooming preparations are sometimes referred to as cosmetics that relax the body. A soothing bath oil can indeed be comforting, and a shampoo session at the hairdresser can be as relaxing as two weeks on the psychiatrist's couch for most women. A great many of the fairer sex admit to keeping their regular weekly date at the beauty shop more for psychological reasons than for the sake of their hair.

If being clean is so important, why not enjoy going about the business of everyday grooming? Treat yourself to a collection of relaxing beauty aids that will make you glad to be as fresh as a rosebud.

Don't just bathe—soak in a scented bath and enjoy the fragrance that will linger with you throughout the day. Use a hair dressing regularly during those dry seasons when your hair is so difficult to keep tame and mannerly. And while you're about it, don't forget Grandma's rule about brushing—do it regularly, and with vigor. Remember, too, that hair suffers a lot more abuse today than in earlier times (although there were periods when it was made to look like a birdcage). It is frequently colored, teased, sprayed, and waved until it hardly remembers its pristine state. Oftentimes the water in which it is washed is extremely hard, and the air in which it lives is full of particles of one unclean sort or another.

Always keep legs and underarms smooth and free of hair. No matter where the hemlines are, or whether sleeves are long or short, *you* know this grooming step is a part of feeling really clean and neat. And if you don't *feel* it, you certainly won't *look* it.

Deodorants and anti-perspirants are made to be used daily, which is precisely what you should do with them.

From after-breakfast brushing with a good dentifrice to the nighttime stint with your toothbrush, you want to feel and appear fresh and clean. There is a world of wonderful cosmetic preparations that make you feel exactly this way.

Cosmetics for grooming purposes can play a part in one of the most pleasurable experiences a woman can have—a time of relaxing and a time devoted to self.

Over the years, those who have recognized the damaging effects of the busy, cluttered world that is woman's, have advised a time of aloneness each day, one spent in refreshing mind and body. Fortunate is the woman who can schedule a whole hour for herself. Actually, this isn't as difficult as one might imagine at first, for surely there is an hour (in total) during the day that can be "borrowed" from time wasted at one thing or another.

With the thought that grooming is important, that

cleanliness is essential, and that an hour devoted to self is positively mind-saving (if not life-extending), give a regular grooming schedule a try.

Begin this glamorous routine by brushing yesterday's spray out of your hair. If a quick re-setting is necessary, dampen hair or spray lightly and set in rollers.

Next, spend fifteen luxurious minutes soaking in a tub that is extravagantly laced with a fragrant oil or filled chin-high with pink bubbles. Work on the mind while you are soaking—read Chaucer in Middle English (or, if you prefer, something not quite so challenging). A brisk rubdown will remove dry skin, and a careful creaming of elbows, legs, and feet will make you feel new all over.

Apply a foundation cream to face and neck: then, snuggled in a warm terry towel or robe, repair your manicure (don't forget the lower ten—feet count, too). Next, take time to make up your face. Enjoy not hurrying during this special hour. Last of all arrange (a euphemism for cussing over and fussing with) your hair.

Voila! Whether or not you *are* truly beautiful, you look it and feel it. Psychologically, the routine is great for clearing mental cobwebs, for restoring confidence, and for making you purr about nearly everything.

Best of all is that you can make most grooming preparations in your kitchen, with fragrances and colors to suit your most personal moods and hours.

HAIR PREPARATIONS

SHAMPOOS are based on soaps or on synthetic soaps (detergents). They should lather well and clean both the hair and the scalp. Those based on soap have the advantage of not removing all the natural oils from the hair; however, they have the disadvantage of reacting with calcium and magnesium salts in water and dulling the hair. Those based on synthetics actually "degrease" the hair and leave it dry and brittle.

To eliminate the dulling effect of soap, lemon juice or vinegar may be added to water to form a rinse. And, if a synthetic is used, see that the shampoo itself has added lanolin or follow shampooing with a lanolin-rich conditioner.

HAIR CONDITIONERS are used to deposit a film of conditioning agents on the hair. They are applied to the hair and distributed thoroughly over the fibers, allowed to remain in contact with the fibers for a brief period, then are rinsed out. We prefer a hot-oil conditioner, used prior to shampooing.

Since most modern shampoos are based on detergents rather than soaps, hair suffers a loss of its natural oils each time it is shampooed. Use of a soap shampoo now and again as well as an oil conditioning treatment, helps restore elasticity and fight dry, brittle hair.

MOUTH PREPARATIONS

Mouth preparations are important grooming aids. Clean teeth and sweet-smelling breath have a great deal to say about us. Here again, general health condition has a significant influence, for decaying teeth or unhealthy gums are not going to be improved very much by being made more fragrant.

TOOTH PASTES AND POWDERS keep the surface of the teeth as clean and shiny as possible, preserve the health of the teeth and gums, and inhibit the formation of unpleasant odors in the mouth. Powders are the simplest tooth cleansers. They can consist only of an abrasive, a wetting agent, and a flavor. Toothpastes contain the same active ingredients as powders, are more expensive to make and more complicated to prepare. However, most people prefer them, probably because their consistency is attractive and they are so convenient to use.

Both pastes and powders are good cleansers and meet the basic requirements of a dentifrice—they must clean without scratching, must not be toxic, and must be refreshing. The choice between paste and powder is entirely one of personal (and usually aesthetic) preference.

MOUTHWASHES have their own role to play in grooming. While tooth pastes and powders act as deodorants as well as cleaning agents, they do not replace the use of mouthwashes. These refreshing liquids reach not only the surface of the teeth but the entire oral cavity as well. Too, they are easy to use and can be carried along to the office or wherever for a pleasant swish now and then during the day.

Flavors, disinfectants, and drug extracts are the important ingredients used in mouthwashes. The final product is often colored with vegetable dye (saffron, carmine, phloxine, erythrosine); however, the dye has no affect on the action of the mouthwash.

DEODORANTS AND ANTI-PERSPIRANTS

DEODORANTS are preparations that not only mask body odor but reduce its intensity. Body odors are caused by the effect of bacteria on apocrine sweat; deodorants act to destroy those odors so that they are not noticed.

Modern deodorants are, in part, based on the toilet-water preparations of the seventeenth-century which persons of means sloshed on themselves to hide odors. Even the ancient Romans were conscious of the need to stay nice-to-be-near—perhaps because they made it their business to be near so many.

ANTI-PERSPIRANTS serve to check perspiration as well as odors. They consist of an aluminum salt, a strong astringent that coagulates proteins, destroys bacteria, and, by constriction of the pores, serves to reduce perspiration secretion.

BATH PREPARATIONS

Bath oils and bubble baths, both products for happier moments a-tubbing, are among the simpler cosmetic formulations you can make for yourself and are also among the "most favorite" gifts from your kitchen.

BUBBLE BATH POWDERS, in addition to the usual bath salt ingredients, contain large amounts of foaming agents in powder form. Most powders soften water, making soap more effective and thus act as aids to hygiene. They may be delicately colored and attractively packaged in tall glass containers.

BATH OILS, because they are insoluble in water, spread as a thin layer on top of the bath. They are *adsorbed* on the skin, making it soft and supple, and their fragrance clings to the skin for hours. These oils, however, do not aid in cleansing; rather, they tend to inhibit lathering. Still, their relaxing effects make them favorites among grooming products. (We are referring to psychological, not medicinal effects.)

HAIR PREPARATIONS

Liquid Shampoo

This is an efficient, simple-to-make shampoo for normal hair.

Tween 80	*1 teaspoon*
Distilled water	*1/3 cup*
Sodium lauryl sulfate or	
ammonium lauryl sulfate	*1 tablespoon*

Mix together all ingredients, heating if necessary to make a smooth solution. *Yield: 1/2 cup.*

Cream Shampoo

This lanolin-enriched shampoo foams beautifully while cleaning efficiently. During the stirring/cooling process it passes through a number of stages, at one point looking for all the world like pizza cheese. But be patient—it finally becomes a beautiful cream.

Sodium hydroxide *	*6 pellets* or
	2/3 of 1/4 teaspoon
Distilled water	*1/4 cup plus 2 tablespoons*
Sodium lauryl sulfate	*1/2 cup*
Lanolin	*1/2 teaspoon*
Stearic acid	*2 teaspoons*

* Sodium hydroxide, traditionally a component of soaps, is a strong caustic. Handle it with care and respect. Whether in dry pellet form or in solution, it must be considered a potentially hazardous material. If the material comes into contact with the skin, immediately flood the area with water until the caustic is washed away, then wash with soap and water.

If the material should splatter into the eye, flush profusely with water and notify a physician immediately about the problem.

Although sodium and potassium hydroxide are extremely corrosive chemicals, they have been commonly used in toilet bowl cleaners for many years. They can be safely used if caution and common sense are employed.

Sodium and potassium hydroxide pellets are hygroscopic, which means they take on moisture from the air. When this occurs, the pellets will stick together. Keep your container of pellets tightly closed to avoid this problem.

Add sodium hydroxide to water. Warm to 158°F (70°C), and add the sodium lauryl sulfate, while stirring. Place lanolin and stearic acid in second beaker and heat to same temperature. Add melted fats to water mixture, with stirring. Stir to room temperature.   *Yield: 1 cup.*

Simple Oil Shampoo

Shampoo advertisements have conditioned us to expect that the excellence of a shampoo is directly proportional to the amount of suds it forms. Suds, television commercials notwithstanding, are not the whole show. A shampoo can be a fine cleaning preparation and one that leaves the hair in young condition even though it doesn't look like foam from Murphy's brew while it is doing its work.

The thing to remember about a shampoo such as this one is that you need to rinse well. It is made primarily of sulfonated oils which are effective detergents, and which can act as conditioning agents.

Sulfonated olive oil	*2 tablespoons*
Sulfonated castor oil	*2 tablespoons*
Distilled water	*1/2 cup*
Color (food coloring), as desired	
Perfume, as desired	

Stir together until well blended. Bottle.   *Yield: 3/4 cup.*

When pellets dissolve in water, an exothermic reaction takes place, that is, the resultant solution will get warm. This kind of solution should be prepared and allowed to cool to room temperature before using.

If at all possible, have the druggist prepare these solutions for you. It will save a lot of wear, tear, and worry.

Soap Shampoo

Why bother with a soap shampoo when there are so many zingy detergent shampoos around? Because a soap shampoo is a refreshing, life-giving treat for dry, brittle hair. Detergent shampoos can strip the hair of its natural oils; soap shampoos will not. However, a soap shampoo will leave a dull film on the hair, which should be removed by using a rinse after shampooing: vinegar and water for brunettes, lemon juice and water for blondes.

This is a formulation for the stout at heart. If you want to prepare an old-fashioned, really fine shampoo, you will consider the project as time well spent.

Potassium hydroxide solution (36%) *	*2 teaspoons*
Coconut oil	*1 tablespoon*
Olive oil	*1 teaspoon*
Castor oil	*1 teaspoon*
Potassium carbonate	*pinch*
Glycerin	*1 teaspoon*
Distilled water	*1/4 cup*

Heat the potassium hydroxide solution in the top of a double boiler to 140°F (60°C). In a separate pan heat coconut, olive, and castor oils to the same temperature. Add

* Ask your druggist to prepare your 36% solution of potassium hydroxide for you. This material is a strong caustic, and your druggist is better qualified and better equipped to prepare it. Don't let this warning keep you from making soap shampoo, soaps have been made for years with animal fats and caustic soda—sodium and/or potassium hydroxide. Please read and heed the warnings included with the formula for Cream Shampoo. Avoid letting potassium hydroxide come in contact with the skin or the eyes.

the potassium hydroxide solution to the oils in a thin stream, stirring continuously. This mixture will get warmer due to the reaction between the hydroxide and oils.

Set aside, covered, until the mixture cools to room temperature. Stir occasionally.

Your soap preparation should end up being *slightly* basic (as opposed to acidic). In order to make sure that it is, you must first make it acidic. Then, by adding sodium hydroxide a little at a time, turn it into a slightly basic solution.

You will need both red and blue litmus papers to test your preparation. An acid solution is detectable because it turns blue litmus red, or because it allows red litmus to stay red, so let's refer to this as "testing red." A basic solution turns red litmus blue or allows blue litmus to stay blue—"testing blue."

Dip a clean table knife into your mixture. Lay a piece of litmus on the cream that clings to the knife after you remove it. If it tests red, you know you have an acidic mixture and you can go ahead to turn it to basic. If your test indicates blue, you know you have a basic situation already, but you don't know just *how* basic, so you must turn it to an acidic preparation as a starting point.

To create the acidic mixture (if you don't already have one), add 1/4 teaspoon of coconut oil to the mixture, wait thirty minutes and test again. Repeat this process until the test is red.

To go to a slightly basic mixture, add 3 drops of sodium hydroxide solution to the now acidic mixture. Wait thirty minutes and test. If you get a blue reaction, your preparation is where it should be. If it still tests red, repeat this process until you get a blue indication.

Now you are in the home stretch. Dissolve potassium carbonate in water and stir into soap. Add glycerin when the mixture is nearly cold. Place in the freezer for a week or so, then remove, allow to come to room temperature. Perfume and package. *Yield: 1/2 cup.*

Hot Oil Conditioner

This simple to make and effective preparation treats dry, brittle hair. Allow enough time in your shampoo schedule to massage scalp with warmed oils and to have a twenty-minute "steaming period" under hot towels. Be certain to shampoo *thoroughly* after towels are removed.

Castor oil	*2 tablespoons*
Olive oil	*1 tablespoon*

Warm oils together in top of double boiler. When they reach a temperature which is comfortable for use, remove from heat and apply immediately to scalp and hair. *Yield: 1/8 cup.*

Hair-Set Preparation

This formula has been around for many years, and is still one of the best setting preparations you can use—store-bought or homemade.

Distilled water	*1/3 cup*
Gum tragacanth	*1/4 teaspoon*
Alcohol	*2 teaspoons*
Glycerin	*1 teaspoon*
Color (food coloring), as desired	
Perfume, as desired	

Warm the water, then sprinkle gum tragacanth on heated water and stir until dissolved. Add remaining ingredients, stirring until well blended. Allow to thicken overnight. *Yield: 1/2 cup.*

MOUTH PREPARATIONS

Toothpaste

If there are youngsters in the home who must be reminded when it is tooth-brushing time, let them make this fine tooth paste and "design" their own flavoring. It's an idea guaranteed to change *their* ideas about brushing!

Milk of magnesia	*1 tablespoon plus 2 teaspoons*
Precipitated chalk	*1 tablespoon plus 1/4 teaspoon*
White powder soap	*1/4 teaspoon*
Gum tragacanth	*1/4 teaspoon*
Glycerin	*2 teaspoons*
Distilled water	*2 teaspoons*
Saccharin	*1 tablet, crushed*
Mineral oil	*1/4 teaspoon*
Flavor, as desired	

Put dry ingredients into mortar and rub down well. Add liquids and rub until smooth paste is obtained. *Yield: 1/4 cup.*

Tooth Powder

This old-fashioned tooth powder is a simple to make, efficient cleanser.

Precipitated chalk (*calcium carbonate*)	*1 3/4 teaspoons*
Magnesium carbonate	*1 teaspoon*
Powdered sugar	*3/4 teaspoon*
Sodium perborate	*1/2 teaspoon*
Powdered neutral white soap	*1/4 teaspoon*
Flavor, as desired	

Put all ingredients except flavoring into mortar and rub down well. Add flavor slowly and continue to rub well until evenly mixed. *Yield: 1/8 cup.*

Mouthwash

Refreshing and sparkling, this preparation will keep your mouth fresh from early morning until well into the day. Experiment with flavorings to add a touch of uniqueness.

Thymol	scant *pinch*
Alcohol * (*vodka*)	*1 teaspoon*
Borax	*1/4 teaspoon*
Sodium bicarbonate	*1/4 teaspoon*
Glycerin	*2 1/2 teaspoons*
Distilled water	*1/3 cup*
Flavor, as desired	
Color, as desired	

Dissolve thymol in alcohol. Dissolve borax, sodium bicarbonate, and glycerin in water. Warm, if necessary to help

* *Do not* use denatured alcohol for any preparation to be taken orally or to be used in the mouth (see Appendix A).

blending. Mix the two solutions, add flavoring (peppermint oil is a good standard), and pour into bottle. *Yield: 1/2 cup.*

DEODORANTS AND ANTI-PERSPIRANTS

Anti-perspirant Cream

This anti-perspirant serves to check perspiration and, at the same time, to prevent unpleasant odor caused by perspiration. It is a pleasantly textured cream.

Synthetic spermaceti wax	*1 teaspoon*
Arlacel 165	*1 tablespoon plus 1 teaspoon*
Sodium lauryl sulfate	*1 teaspoon*
Aluminum sulfate	*2 teaspoons*
Distilled water	*3 tablespoons*
Glycerin	*3/4 teaspoon*
Perfume, as desired	

Heat spermaceti wax, Arlacel 165, and Sodium lauryl sulfate in top of double boiler to a temperature of 158°F (70°C). In a second double boiler heat aluminum sulfate, water, and glycerin to same temperature and add, slowly and while stirring, to first mixture. Stir to 86°F (30°C), add perfume, and pour into jar. *Yield: 1/2 cup.*

Liquid Anti-perspirant

Those who prefer a liquid anti-perspirant to a cream will enjoy making and using this formula. It is an effective deodorant and anti-perspirant.

Aluminum chloride	*1 1/4 teaspoons*
Urea	*3/4 teaspoon*
Glycerin	*1/2 teaspoon*
Distilled water	*1/3 cup*
Color (food coloring), as desired	
Perfume (water soluble), as desired	

This is a simple solution. Pour all ingredients into container and shake until dissolved.

A suggestion: package in a plastic spray bottle (available at drug and dime stores) or plunger-type spray bottle. *Yield: 1/3 cup.*

BATH PREPARATIONS

Foam Bath

This luxurious, frothy bath treat makes an especially nice gift for the youngsters on your list.

Triethanolamine lauryl sulfate	*3 tablespoons*
Borax	*1/2 teaspoon*
Distilled water	*3 tablespoons*
Color, as desired	
Perfume, as desired	

Simply mix the ingredients. Swirl until the borax is dissolved. Add a drop of food coloring and perfume to suit. *Yield: 1/3 cup.*

Bath Oil

Bath oils are among the oldest cosmetics. Using them creates the most luxurious, relaxing moments during a grooming routine. This is an extremely simple, and very pleasing, preparation.

Tween 20	*2 tablespoons*
Distilled water	*1/2 cup*
Perfume, as desired	*up to 1 teaspoon*

Stir together all ingredients until well blended.   *Yield: 2/3 cup.*

Bath Salts

Each of the following materials is an effective, attractive water softener for the bath.

Sodium carbonate or

Sodium sesquicarbonate or

Borax

Place any one of the above in a quart jar, filling jar less than half-full. Add several drops of perfume, place lid on jar, and shake vigorously until perfume oil appears to be evenly dispersed. Repeat with one or two drops of food coloring. Package in desired containers. Note: Borax is less soluble than the other materials, so add it to the bath early, allowing more time for it to dissolve.

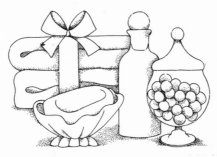

Add about two tablespoons of bath salts to a tub of water. You may prefer to use more, or less, but this amount is average for most users.

Body Oil

If you don't treat yourself to a body rub with a blend of rich oils at least once in your life, you have missed something that women have delighted in since centuries before Cleopatra first tried it.

Since you are obviously going to be deliciously oily, guard against soiling sheets (if you plan to leave the oils on until your morning tub) or furniture.

An all-over oil treatment affects the entire body almost as positively as it does the psyche. Experiment with the combinations of oils you find most pleasing. The following is a good place to begin:

Sesame oil	*1 tablespoon*
Wheat-germ oil	*1 tablespoon*
Avocado oil	*1 tablespoon*
Perfume oil, as desired	

Stir together until well blended, then bottle. *Yield: 1/4 cup.*

11

There's a Man in the Kitchen

Anyone who isn't excited by the new men's colognes and the scents of modern shaving preparations has to be either too young or too old. While the psychology of fragrance has become interesting study for a number of researchers, certain aspects of the phenomenon require only laboratory observation. Put a man wearing one of the jungle or island scents (actually, the scents are named to create atmosphere—nobody's going to buy essence of jungle) into a crowd of women and watch them respond. End of experiment.

There is no denying the great new interest in cosmetics for men. No self-respecting hero of spy thrillers would pass up an opportunity to have a new after-shave named after him, and a fringe benefit of professional sports is endorsing men's cosmetics.

Cosmetics for men, if we believe what we read in advertisements, have to be *totally* and *unquestionably* for men. They have to bring out the beast in a fellow and desire in his woman. They have got to have guts and gusto or they are not masculine enough for the man's side of the medicine cabinet. For some reason, it seems that such items as hairsprays and deodorants cannot be unisex products, although certain manufacturers have tried a "for the entire family" approach to selling cosmetics. Their success is debatable.

All of which is to say that men's cosmetics have come into their own. Men are buying and using more grooming (and beautifying) products than at any time in *modern* history. Records of the past tell us that men, from time to time, have been more interested in cosmetics than women have, painting and powdering and perfuming to the point where they probably were nicer to be away from than close to.

With this current interest in cosmetics, it is the wise man who "cooks" the preparations he uses, making them fit the personality that is his and seeing that they please the women who please him.

Does a man belong on the end of a stirring rod in the kitchen? Indeed he does. Men are naturals at creating, born do-it-yourselfers. Making cosmetics is fun for the man of the house who is bored silly with the same old hobby he has had since the day his neighbor talked him into woodworking.

While packing hair lacquers and he-man deodorants into aerosol cans isn't appropriate for kitchen concocting, there are still many great cosmetics for men that can be made at home—and made by men.

Good things that men can make for themselves and the fellows who make up their Saturday morning golf foursomes include shaving creams, before-shave and after-shave lotions, hair preparations, zinc oxide ointment (for the outdoor sportsman), colognes, perfumes, and deodorants. Also, a rich, salve-like hand lubricating cream is a lemon-scented blessing for most men, and it is a wonderfully satisfactory homemade cosmetic.

Experiment with fragrances for men's cosmetics— the druggist has some good scents to try (bay rum, lemon, lime, orange, and the like). Remember that fragrances and flavors used in cosmetics are concentrated; don't try using brandy or bourbon, for the fragrance and flavor are lost. However, brandy or bourbon *flavoring* can be used for the man who has special tastes along these lines.

And so, men, have at it. Cosmetic chemistry can be a man's game (and usually is). As a hobby, it beats hammers and nails.

HAIR PREPARATIONS

As men's hairstyles change, so does the need for hairdressings. During the crewcut stage, men had little need for a product to keep the hair gleaming and manageable. In the 1970's, men's hairstyles have gone to new lengths —sometimes even to the shoulders. This means that a good hairdressing is essential if the hair is to be kept neat and well groomed.

Different kinds of hairdressings have been "in" during different periods. During the Clark Gable–Tyrone Power era (and even earlier) the look in vogue was smooth and slick. More recently, men and boys have objected strongly to the "greasy kid-stuff" kind of preparation, and hairdressings promising a natural look while controlling the hair have become extremely popular.

The principal purpose of most hairdressings is to hold the hair in place and to make it lustrous. Also, hairdressings fight dry, brittle hair and give it a healthier appearance.

There is a wide variety of hair preparations on the market. Some you can make conveniently in your kitchen.

SHAVING PREPARATIONS

The man who shaves with a blade understands that there is more to shaving creams and lotions than aesthetic value. To the man who shaves with an electric razor, the use of a pre-shave or after-shave lotion may appear to be more for psychological effect than for anything else. However, even with an electric razor, preparing the skin for an attack on the beard can make shaving more comfortable and more efficient. With a blade, the use of some kind of pre-shave preparation is essential.

Soaps, creams, or lotions applied to the skin before shaving help to soften the skin's surface, make the hair stand erect (and thus easier to cut), and help the cutting edge glide smoothly on the skin.

After-shave preparations make the skin feel refreshed

and create a pleasant kind of tingling sensation. They contain alcohol, water, perfume, and an astringent. Some contain a mild antiseptic.

How the skin is affected by shaving depends upon many factors involved in this daily grooming chore: the condition of skin and hair, the shaving technique, the sharpness of the blade or the construction of the razor, etc. Regardless, it's a fact of a man's life that a certain amount of skin irritation cannot be avoided in the shaving process. The top layer of the stratum corneum has been scraped, and, especially if a blade is used, the skin sometimes suffers a multitude of tiny, non-bleeding cuts.

Shaving lotions are designed to relieve the undesirable side-effects of scraping the epidermis.

HAND PREPARATIONS

While a man may use any kind of hand cream or lotion to soften and protect the skin, frequently the nature of his work (or play) means extra-dry, rough skin that needs a special kind of treatment. A salve-like lubricating cream rich in lanolin is an especially important cosmetic for men. Used regularly, it softens and protects. Too, if it is applied generously at night, it has a chance to work on the hands undisturbed, serving as a treatment for dry skin.

Special hand cleaners work at removing dirt and grime from masculine hands, a good place to begin for regular hand care.

CREAMS

Use of skin creams is not limited to women. Men also use creams, but for different reasons than women do. Usually when a man applies a cream to his skin he does so because he wants to protect or soothe it; he is not interested in fighting wrinkles or making himself more beautiful.

Two kinds of creams enjoyed by men are protective skin creams (for those hours spent on the golf course or in a fishing boat) and mentholated massage creams. Formulas are included for both of these.

DEODORANTS

Most men are aware of the need for regular use of an effective deodorant. Many of them find a stick deodorant aesthetically more pleasing than a spray, cream, or roll-on preparation. Included below is an excellent deodorant in stick form, pleasant to use and effective at fighting body odor.

PERFUMES FOR MEN

What kind of men use perfumes? The usual kind.

History tells us that men have always used perfumes. Pleasant scents have great influence on those sniffing them, and there is no telling how important a splash of perfume might have been at a crucial moment in the course of world history.

There is no reason to think that men must be *au naturel* when it comes to scent. Essence of cigar smoke doesn't have to be the *only* fragrance associated with masculinity.

There are fragrances that have been designed specifically to please men. For hundreds of years men have favored scents created from a variety of fragrant balsams, enjoying perfumes such as the chypres and "leathers" and other good concoctions pleasing to male nostrils and imaginations.

Experiment with scents for men. Included is a formula for a men's cologne; however, the actual perfume to be used is left to the formulator. Try buying perfume concentrates from the druggist, then blend them (or use them straight) to make the cologne something special.

See "Preparations to Beautify" (pp. 76–106) for instructions on making homemade perfumes from scratch. The same technique can be used in making perfumes to scent men's cologne, or to make finished perfumes for men.

HAIR PREPARATIONS

Hair Cream

This cream is typical of best-sellers on the men's cosmetic counter. It tames the hair, keeps it in place, and does good things without effecting a slicked-down look.

Petrolatum	2 teaspoons
Mineral oil	1 tablespoon plus 2 teaspoons
Lanolin	3/4 teaspoon
Arlacel 165	1 teaspoon
Beeswax	1/2 teaspoon
Borax	pinch
Water	3 tablespoons
Perfume, as desired	

Heat petrolatum, mineral oil, lanolin, Arlacel 165, and beeswax in top of double boiler to a temperature of 158°F (70°C). Heat borax and water to the same temperature and add to first mixture. Beat slowly with an egg beater until the mixture reaches 104°F (40°C). Perfume may be added if desired. Pour into jar. *Yield: 1/3 cup.*

Clear Hairdressing

A simple, yet totally satisfactory preparation to keep hair tame and well behaved.

| G-1790 | 1 tablespoon |
| Distilled water | 1/3 cup plus 1 tablespoon |

Heat the G-1790 to 158°F (70°C). Heat the water to the same temperature and add to G-1790. Stir until cool. *Yield: 1/2 cup.*

SHAVING PREPARATIONS

Brushless Shaving Cream No. 1

Brushless shaving creams do not lather very much (if at all), but keep the beard moist and erect to help the razor to move smoothly (and painlessly) over the skin.

Stearic acid	*1 tablespoon*
Propylene glycol monostearate	*3/4 teaspoon*
Mineral oil	*3/4 teaspoon*
Glycerin	*1 teaspoon*
Triethanolamine	*1/4 teaspoon*
Distilled water	*1/3 cup*

Heat stearic acid, propylene glycol monostearate, and mineral oil in top of double boiler to a temperature of 167°F (75°C). Heat the rest of the ingredients to the same temperature in a second double boiler, then add to first mixture slowly and with stirring. Stir while cooling and pour into jar. *Yield: 1/2 cup.*

Brushless Shaving Cream No. 2

Lanolin enriches this efficient, very pleasing brushless shaving cream.

Mineral oil	*1/4 teaspoon*
Cetyl alcohol	*1/2 teaspoon*
Lanolin	*1/2 teaspoon*
Stearic acid	*1 tablespoon plus 1 teaspoon*
Triethanolamine	*1/4 teaspoon*
Borax	*pinch*
Distilled water	*1/4 cup*
Glycerin	*1 3/4 teaspoons*
Perfume, as desired	

Heat mineral oil, cetyl alcohol, lanolin, and stearic acid to a temperature of 167°F (75°C) in a double boiler. In a second double boiler, heat the glycerin, triethanolamine, water, and borax to a temperature of 176°F (80°C), then add to first mixture, while stirring. Continue slow stirring until the material is almost cooled. Perfume oil is then stirred in carefully. The cream should be left to stand overnight in a glass or earthenware container. Stir it once again the next day, then put in an appropriate container.　*Yield: 1/2 cup.*

Electric Pre-shave Lotion

Even when an electric razor is used, it is well to prepare the skin for the daily shaving chore.

Alcohol	*1/4 cup*
Sorbo	*1 teaspoon*
Menthol	scant *pinch*
Water	*1/4 cup*
Perfume, as desired	
Color (food coloring), as desired	

Dissolve menthol in alcohol, then add other ingredients and stir until clear. Add perfume and food coloring as desired. *Yield: 1/2 cup.*

After-shave Stick

Deliciously refreshing and cooling, this preparation is certain to please the man making it (and the friends he makes it for). It forms a beautiful, translucent stick.

Stearic acid	*1 teaspoon*
Sorbo	*1/2 teaspoon*
Alcohol	*1/3 cup plus 2 tablespoons*
Sodium hydroxide *	*5 pellets*
Distilled water	*1 teaspoon*
Menthol	scant *pinch*
Perfume, *as desired*	

Heat stearic acid, Sorbo, and alcohol in top of double boiler to a temperature of 149°F (65°C). Heat sodium hydroxide and water to a temperature of 158°F (70°C), then add to first mixture, while stirring. Remove from heat and continue stirring to 131–140°F (55–60°C). Add menthol and perfume, then pour into mold and allow to cool slowly.

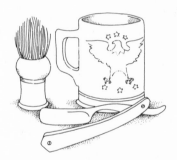

MAKING THE MOLD: Wrap aluminum foil around a candle, about 3/4 inch in diameter. Carefully fold bottom ends under. The finished mold should be of at least two thicknesses, and about four inches high. To assure that there will be no leakage during cooling, light the candle when you remove it and drip a thin layer of wax on the bottom of the mold.   *Yield: 1/2 cup.*

* See remarks on pp. 115–16 concerning use of sodium hydroxide, an ingredient which can be hazardous when used improperly.

After-shave Lotion

There's a lot of zing and zest in this after-shave lotion with guaranteed "wake-up" power. It leaves the skin feeling smooth and refreshed.

Witch hazel	*1 tablespoon*
Alcohol	*1 tablespoon*
Menthol crystals *	scant *pinch*
Alum	*pinch*
Boric acid	*1/4 teaspoon*
Glycerin	*1 teaspoon*
Distilled water	*1/4 cup plus 1 teaspoon*

Mix witch hazel, alcohol, and menthol in a container.. Heat alum, boric acid, glycerin, and water in the top of a double boiler until alum and boric acid are dissolved. Allow to cool, then mix the two solutions, stir, and package.   *Yield: 1/2 cup.*

HAND PREPARATIONS

Extra-rich Hand Lubricant

This cream, almost like a salve, is smooth and glossy, a rich lubricating product that will soften very dry skin. It will feel greasy on the hands, and is best used at night

---

* You may reduce (or eliminate) the menthol and use bay rum or another suitable perfume.

before retiring. For those doing rough work, this product is a godsend!

Boric acid	*1 1/2 teaspoons*
Glycerin	*3 tablespoons plus 1/2 teaspoon*
Lanolin	*1/4 cup*
Petrolatum	*1/3 cup plus 1 tablespoon plus 1 teaspoon*
Perfume, as desired	

Warm boric acid and glycerin in top of double boiler over water until dissolved. Allow to cool. Place the lanolin and petrolatum in a small mixing bowl and blend with a spatula until the mixture is smooth and creamy. Next, add the mixture of boric acid and glycerin, little by little, working it into the lanolin mixture.

Lanolin has a characteristic odor that is rather unpleasant. We like to work in a healthy amount of lemon oil (USP) along with the glycerin and boric acid mixture. It imparts a fresh, lemony fragrance to the finished product. You may prefer to use another USP oil.   *Yield: 1 cup.*

Hand Cleaner No. 1

Waterless hand cleaner is a wonderful preparation for a man whose work and hobbies mean that he meets lots of dirt and grime. It forms a thick paste, which is the way it goes on the hands. Water is added and it immediately foams and goes to work. You can effect changes in consistency by experimenting with this formula.

Lanolin	3/4 teaspoon
Glycerin	1 tablespoon
Detergent (sodium lauryl sulfate) *	1 tablespoon plus 1 teaspoon
Kaolin **	2 tablespoons
Perfume, as desired	

Heat lanolin and glycerin until lanolin has melted, using a double boiler. Add detergent and kaolin and mix thoroughly. Perfume as desired.   *Yield: 1/3 cup.*

Hand Cleaner No. 2

Pumice in this hand cleaner makes it more abrasive and harder working than the waterless hand cleaner. Give them both a try to see which you prefer.

Glycerin	1/2 teaspoon
Borax	1 teaspoon
Sodium carbonate	1/2 teaspoon
Distilled water	1/3 cup
Powdered soap	2 teaspoons
Pumice	1 tablespoon

Dissolve glycerin, borax, and sodium carbonate in about 1/3 of the water. Dissolve the soap in the remaining water, then mix the two solutions. Add pumice, stirring continuously, as mixture thickens.   *Yield: 1/2 cup.*

---

* You may use a liquid detergent, such as a dishwashing liquid, in which case you should eliminate or reduce the glycerin.
** You may use pumice instead of kaolin for a more abrasive cleaner.

d to the skin, has a feeling more refreshing than
ohol-based preparations. Jazz it up with a scent you
 especially interesting. You may even want to de-
 your own by using a combination of perfume oils
ilable from your druggist.

Tween 20	*1 tablespoon plus 1 teaspoon*
Distilled water	*1/3 cup*
Perfume concentrate	*1 teaspoon*

ce in tightly closed container and shake. *Yield: 1/2*

CREAMS

Protective Sun Cream

For those who enjoy outdoor sports, a protective cream
is almost a necessity. This cream protects noses that
spend lots of time on fishing boats, skis, golf courses, or
wherever.

Beeswax	*1 teaspoon*
Petrolatum	*1/4 cup*
Mineral oil	*1 tablespoon plus 1 teaspoon*
Zinc oxide	*1 teaspoon*

Heat beeswax and petroleum in top of double boiler to a
temperature of 167°F (75°C). Stir when melted. Place mineral oil and zinc oxide in mortar and work well. Add the
melted wax mixture when it drops in temperature to about
104°F (40°C). Mix thoroughly, and place in jar. *Yield:*
1/3 cup.

Mentholated Cream for Massage

If this cream can't cure muscle fatigue, it certainly can
make a tired body feel better. It is a boon for aching
muscles, pleasing to use, and very effective.

Stearic acid	*1 tablespoon plus 1 teaspoon*
Lanolin	*1/2 teaspoon*
Glycerin	*1 teaspoon*
Triethanolamine	*1/4 teaspoon*
Distilled water	*1/4 cup*
Menthol	*1/4 teaspoon*
Methyl salicylate	*2 teaspoons*

Melt stearic acid and lanolin in top of double boiler, heating to a temperature of 176°F (80°C). In a second double boiler heat glycerin, triethanolamine, and water to the same temperature, then add to stearic acid and lanolin, while stirring. Remove from heat and immediately add menthol and methyl salicylate. Continue vigorous stirring until cool. Package as you would a cold cream.   *Yield: 1/2 cup.*

DEODORANTS

Deodorant Stick

Deodorant sticks are great cosmetics for the man's side of the bathroom cabinet. They are pleasing to use and work very well at the job of keeping him nice to be near.

Petrolatum	2 tablespoons
Paraffin wax	1 1/2 teaspoons
Synthetic spermaceti wax	1 tablespoon plus 2 teaspoons
Beeswax	1 tablespoon
Aluminum chloride or zinc peroxide	1/2 teaspoon
Zinc oxide	1/2 teaspoon
Zinc stearate	1 tablespoon
Perfume, as desired	

In top of double boiler heat petrolatum, paraffin wax, spermaceti wax, and beeswax to a temperature of 167°F (75°C). Place the aluminum chloride, zinc oxide, and zinc stearate in a mortar and rub down well. Mix the finely ground powders with the warm waxes while stirring. Pour directly into mold while 140°F (60°C) for warmer. Use glass tools when

working with this formula, for alum tack stainless steel and other metals.

For notes on making molds, s panying After-shave Stick on p. 13?

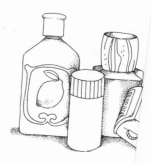

Deodorant Foot Powder

This is the type of powder whic military. It is a wonderful treat and refreshing.

Thymol	1 teaspoon
Boric acid	2 tablespoons
Zinc oxide	1 tablespoon p
Talc	1/4 cup plus 3

Place all ingredients in a mortar 3/4 cup.

PERFUME

Men's Cologne

The fun of making a prepa perimenting with fragrance

kir
alc
fin
sig
ava

Pla
cup

Appendices

Definitions
and
Sources of Supply

ALCOHOL   Denatured ethyl alcohol contains materials which cannot be removed and which make it poison, so don't try drinking it. In formulas calling for alcohol, vodka may be used instead, even though it is only 40–60 percent alcohol. Alcohol acts as a solvent in cosmetics. It also evaporates rapidly, promoting a cooling effect in shaving lotions and similar preparations. Available at drug stores.

ALMOND OIL (sweet)   Both an emollient and a flavoring. Available in drug, food and most health food stores.

ALUM (ammonium aluminum sulfate or potassium aluminum sulfate)   An astringent. It is a cosmetic ingredient that has been used for this purpose for as long as almost anyone can remember. Buy it at the drugstore.

ALUMINUM SULFATE   An astringent, used primarily in deodorants and anti-perspirants. Do not use anything but the pure, reagent grade of aluminum sulfate. Available at the drug store or through a chemical suppy house.

AMBERGRIS   Used in fine perfumes, ambergris is formed in the intestinal tract of the sperm whale. It is most commonly used as a tincture. When it is added to a perfume, its own long-lasting scent enhances the finished product. Ambergris has been used since the days of antiquity, prized as a perfume and as a drug. It is available from suppliers of perfume concentrates.

AMMONIUM ALUMINUM SULFATE (see *Alum*).

ANGELICA   A kind of aromatic herb whose roots and fruit are used to make Angelica oil for perfumes. Artificial Angelica is available for a modest cost. Order it from a supplier of perfume concentrates.

ANTIOXIDANT   Refers to a material that retards oxidation and thus rancidity of a cosmetic preparation.

ARLACELS, SORBO, SPANS, TWEENS   All are emulsifying agents and surfactants. Each has properties making it uniquely suitable for a particular kind of emulsion. Sometimes they work in pairs. The chemical names (listed in order below) sound rather prestigious for the kitchen; however, they work as well there as in the laboratory. They create, through their emulsifying properties, stable, good-looking cosmetic preparations. All of them are manufactured by Atlas Chemical Co. and all can be ordered from Emulsion Engineering, Inc., or Van Waters and Rogers United Co.

ARLACEL 60   Sorbitan monostearate (see *Arlacels*).

ARLACEL 80   Sorbitan monooleate (see *Arlacels*).

ARLACEL 83   Sorbitan sesquioleate (see *Arlacels*).

ARLACEL 165   Glycerol monostearate, acid-stable, self-emulsifying (see *Arlacels*).

ARLACEL 186   Mono and diglycerides of fat-forming fatty acids (see *Arlacels*).

AVOCADO OIL   A good emollient, rich in vitamins and used over the years to soften the skin and lessen problems with facial lines. Available at some drug and most health food stores, it is also available from Calavo Growers of California.

BEESWAX   The product of the digestion of worker bees used in constructing the cell walls of the honeycomb. Its use in cosmetics is historic. Modern formulas use it in combination with borax to form stiff, stable creams. Buy it at drug and hobby stores.

BENTONITE   A colloidal clay obtained from volcanic ash, used in face masks and similar preparations because of its ability to absorb water up to 15 times its own volume. Available at drug stores.

BENZOIN, TINCTURE OF   A balsamic resin, an alcoholic solution of certain benzoins plus additional ingredients. It is used medicinally and in cosmetics as a topical skin protectant. Available at all drug stores.

BERGAMOT OIL, SYNTHETIC   A chemically made substitute for an oil obtained from the skin of the bergamot fruit, a member of the citrus family. Bergamot oil is used extensively in the perfume industry to enhance the fragrance of the finished product. The synthetic oil is available from suppliers of perfume concentrates.

BORAX   A colorless, crystalline, alkali substance that is an excellent cleanser and softens water. With beeswax it forms the beeswax/borax soap which is the basis for many creams. Readily available in drug and food stores.

BORIC ACID   A mild antiseptic. Although it has bactericidal and fungicidal properties, it may be used in cosmetic preparations provided it is used according to formula directions. The powder, as it is packaged, should not be used itself as a cosmetic. Do *not* take it orally! Buy it in drug and some food stores.

BUTYL ACETATE A volatile, active solvent used in nail polishes and nail polish removers. Available at the drug store or from a chemical supply house.

BUTYL STEARATE Provides good adhesion of cream preparations, promoting a softer feeling to the skin. In nail buffing paste it serves to make the product less gritty. Order from a chemical supply house.

CALCIUM CARBONATE (see *Precipitated chalk*).

CARNAUBA WAX Obtained from the leaf of the carnauba palm in Brazil. It imparts stiffness to cosmetic preparations. Buy it in drug, candle, or hobby stores.

CASTOR OIL The oil of the castor bean, has abundant commercial applications, including use in detergents, resins, fibers, and cosmetics. It is a solvent for color pigments. Castor oil has a smooth, glossy shine and is used in lipsticks and hair dressings. Buy it at the drug store.

CASTOR OIL, SULFONATED (turkey red oil) A mild detergent. If your druggist doesn't have it, he can order it from GAF Corp., Welch, Holme and Clark, Inc., or Baker Castor Oil Co. (See also *Olive oil, sulfonated.*)

CERESINE WAX Derived from petroleum and is a specially refined grade of ozokerite. It is a microcrystalline wax which thickens oil mixtures without liquifying under pressure. If your druggist doesn't have it on hand, it can be ordered from Cornelius Wax Co.

CETYL ALCOHOL (1-hexadecanol) In small amounts, improves both the texture and low-temperature stability of creams. It is a white solid which comes as small white flakes. Buy from the drug store or order from a chemical supply house.

CIVET   A glandular secretion from both male and female civet cats. Civet used commercially is produced by cats kept in captivity for that purpose. The material is added to perfumes to enhance their fragrance. It is available from suppliers of perfume concentrates.

COCOA BUTTER   An excellent lubricant and can be used as is for softening the skin. It can also be used for massage and for protection against sun and wind. In formulations it acts as an emollient in soaps and creams. Readily available at the drug store.

COCONUT OIL   Reacts with the alkali in shampoo and similar formulations to form a soap of excellent quality. Readily available at the drug store.

(DI) ETHYLENE GLYCOL MONOETHYL ETHER   A humectant, reducing evaporation and treating the surface of the skin to avoid rough, broken areas. Order from a chemical supply house.

EMOLLIENT   A product for the care of the corneal (outermost) skin layer. It acts to prevent the degreasing or drying out of the corneal layer by lubricating the skin.

EMULSION   A system in which globules of a liquid (the dispersed phase) are held in suspension in another liquid (the continuous phase). When two immiscible (incompatible) liquids such as oil and water are mixed, they tend to separate into distinct layers. Emulsifying agents are materials which surround minute droplets of oil (or water) so that they are held in suspension. There are two basic types of emulsions: O/W (oil in water) and W/O (water in oil).

EPSOM SALT   (see *Magnesium sulfate*).

ESTER   A term used in organic chemistry to describe organic salts. Many of the compounds used in cosmetic chemistry (such as the parabens) are esters.

FLAVORINGS   Your druggist will carry a supply of flavorings for cosmetics. Also investigate your grocery and health food stores.

FLOWER WATERS   Aromatic waters made from volatile oils or other aromatic volatile substances. They are clear, saturated, aqueous solutions frequently used in skin tonics, fresheners, and similar preparations. Examples of flower waters are rose water and orange flower water.

G-1790   Polyoxyethylene lanolin derivative (see *Arlacels*).

G-2162   Polyoxyethylene propylene glycol stearate (see *Arlacels*).

GELATIN   One of the more familiar cosmetic ingredients. Its protein content is well known to women who have taken gelatin for years in an attempt to strengthen nails. It is used in cosmetics primarily for its gelling qualities. Buy *unflavored* gelatin at food stores.

GLYCERYL MONOSTEARATE   Forms neutral creams. It is marketed in both self-emulsifying and non-self-emulsifying grades. Both are excellent emulsifying agents, but the self-emulsifying grade has some soap-making capabilities. Order from a chemical supply house.

GUM TRAGACANTH   (see *Tragacanth, gum*).

HAMAMELIS WATER   (see *Witch hazel*).

HELIOTROPIN   An aromatic chemical used in perfumes to enhance the fragrance of the finished product. It is available from suppliers of perfume concentrates and aromatic chemicals.

HUMECTANT A hygroscopic (water-gathering) material which prevents or lessens shrinkage of cream by reducing evaporation. It smooths skin surface and prevents or cures roughness or breaks in the "horny" layer of the skin. It eases cream application and prevents a "rolling" effect.

1-HEXADECANOL (see *Cetyl alcohol*).

ISOPROPYL MYRISTATE An organic salt used in cosmetics to avoid the sticky, greasy feeling in preparations containing high fat or oil content. Order from a chemical supply house.

JASMINE, ARTIFICIAL A chemically made constituent of many perfumes. Manufacturers strive to approximate the fine sweet odor of the natural jasmine flower by using commercial absolute essences or by carrying out research on the flower itself. Artificial jasmine is available from suppliers of perfume concentrates.

KAOLIN A naturally occurring clay (kaolinite) which is finely ground and specially processed for use in cosmetics. It gives bulk and "slip" and absorbs moisture. Its surface activity and detergent properties make it an important ingredient in face masks. Buy it from your druggist. Ask for colloidal kaolin.

LANOLIN Occupies a special place among animal waxes, for of all the natural raw materials, it is the most similar to human skin and hair fat, both in chemical composition and in physiological properties. It is a valuable ingredient in preparations designed to replace skin fat and to restore or maintain the skin's normal elasticity. It is nontoxic and non-irritating. Ask for *anhydrous* lanolin, but *hydrous* lanolin (a yellow-white, sticky cream) will do if that's all your druggist has in stock. Some formulas also call for liquid lanolin, which your druggist should be able to supply.

LECITHIN   An emollient, is a constituent of the human skin. It is *not* a hormone. In cosmetics it is a thickening agent, similar to gum tragacanth. Buy powdered, not granulated, lecithin from your druggist.

LITMUS PAPER   A chemical test paper. Red litmus indicates an acid solution; blue litmus indicates a basic solution. Available at hobby stores and toy shops that carry chemistry sets.

MAGNESIUM CARBONATE   Used in a wide variety of preparations, but here it is used in toothpaste for its abrasive effect. Your druggist can order it from his supplier, or you can order it from a chemical supply house.

MAGNESIUM SULFATE (epsom salt)   Stabilizes water-in-oil cream emulsions. Buy it at your drug store.

METHYL CELLULOSE   Used as a surfactant and stabilizer for emulsions. It is basically a thickening agent, similar to the gums. Order it from a chemical supply house.

METHYL PARABEN   A widely used cosmetic preservative. Parabens are esters of p-hydroxybenzoic acid, and have been said to approximate the perfect preservative. Either you or your druggist can order it from a chemical supply house.

METHYL SALICYLATE (oil of wintergreen)   A counter-irritant. It has a cooling effect and is absorbed by the skin. It has long been used as an athletic "rub down." Available in all drug stores.

MILK OF MAGNESIA   Used in tooth preparations to help whiten teeth and to assist in removal of stain. It also neutralizes acids in the oral cavity. Available in drug and food stores.

MINERAL OIL (liquid petrolatum)   A mixture of liquid hydrocarbons derived from petroleum. It is widely used in cosmetic products because of its neutral, stable, and odorless character. It softens and protects the skin. Buy it in drug and food stores.

MUSK   The major animal perfume. Animal perfumes are important in the manufacture of finished perfumes, for they enhance the final product by giving it life and diffusiveness. Musk is a dried secretion of the male musk deer. Buy it from any supplier of perfume concentrates. It is also found in some novelty shops.

NEROLI OIL   An essential oil used in perfume making. Artificial Neroli oil is available at a fraction of the cost of the natural oil. Buy it from a supplier of perfume concentrates.

OLEIC ACID   A fatty acid which reacts with the alkali in a formulation to form a soap. Order from a chemical supply house.

OLIVE OIL   An emollient used for centuries because of its softening and lubricating properties, and, practically speaking, because of its almost universal availability. Buy it at food stores.

OLIVE OIL, SULFONATED (turkey red oil)   A mild detergent. It has good wetting and dispersing properties, fair emulsifying and poor foaming effects. It is a cleansing agent. Ask your druggist for the sulfonated oil.

ORANGE FLOWER WATER   (see *Flower waters*).

OZOKERITE   A purified grade of natural mineral waxes. It is a microcrystalline wax which produces a firm cream. If you find a wax called simply "microcrystalline wax," you may assume it is ozokerite. Buy it at drug and hobby stores. It is also available from Cornelius Wax Co.

PARAFFIN WAX   Derived from distillation of petroleum. It is a familiar item in the kitchen, used for home canning. In cosmetics it produces soft creams. It is used in oily mixtures to provide desired *thixotropic* properties. Creams should be firm while in the jar, but should liquify on the skin. Materials that help this change to occur are said to have thixotropic properties. Paraffin wax is readily available at drug, hobby, and food stores.

PERFUME OILS (concentrates) Used to impart fragrances to cosmetic preparations, or to manufacture finished perfumes. Many are available at the drug store. They also may be ordered from such companies as Florasynth Labs, Inc., Norda Essential Oil Co., Synfleur Scientific Labs, Van Dyke and Co.

PETROLATUM (petroleum jelly) A purified mixture of semi-solid hydrocarbons obtained from petroleum, either entirely or partly deodorized. It is used as a lubricant in cosmetics, and is frequently used alone for its soothing, softening properties. For cosmetic use it is necessary to buy *white* petroleum jelly, the purest grade. Available in all drug and most food stores.

PHENYL SALICYLATE CRYSTALS (salol) A reasonably good sun screen. Available at the drug store.

PIGMENTS (cosmetic colors) Your druggist may carry some of the more common pigments, or you can order them through a chemical supply house or manufacturer of cosmetic colorants such as Sun Chemical Co., Florasynth Labs, Inc., Leeben Color and Chemical Co., Whittaker, Clark and Daniels, etc. You will want to write to a colorant manufacturer for catalogs containing color samples so that you will know how to use pigments for makeup preparations. (See comments in "Perfumes, Colors, and Preservatives," pp. 33–39).

POTASSIUM ALUMINUM SULFATE (see *Alum*).

POTASSIUM CARBONATE   Combines with fatty acid ingredients in cosmetics to form mild soaps. Available from the drug store or from a chemical supply house.

PRECIPITATED CHALK (calcium carbonate)   Widely used as an abrasive in tooth paste and powder preparations. In finely powdered form, it is also a good face powder ingredient. Buy it at the drug store.

PROPYLENE GLYCOL   A colorless, odorless liquid resembling glycerin in its properties. It acts as a humectant and serves to inhibit the growth of molds. Order it from a chemical supply house. (In a pinch, glycerin may be substituted for propylene glycol.)

PROPYLENE GLYCOL MONOSTEARATE   An emulsifying agent and surfactant. It is one of those materials that makes beautiful emulsions happen in your kitchen. It can be ordered from a chemical supply house.

ROSE OIL (water soluble)   A scent for water-base cosmetic preparations. Available in drug stores.

ROSE WATER   (see *Flower waters*).

SACCHARIN   A sweetner for preparations for oral use, such as toothpastes. Available in drug and food stores.

SESAME OIL   An excellent emollient, lubricates and softens the skin. It absorbs ultraviolet light well, and is sometimes used in suntan preparations. Health food, drug, and some food stores carry it.

SILICA, POWDERED   An abrasive. Buy it at the drug store.

SOAP, POWDERED (castile)   A pure soap and is used as a cleansing agent. Buy it in the baby products department of the drug store.

SODIUM BICARBONATE, CARBONATE, AND SESQUICARBONATE Used in bath preparations as water softeners and to create effervescent effects. Which of the three is used depends upon availability and aesthetic value. You may substitute one for the other. Buy them in drug and some food stores.

SODIUM LAURYL SULFATE   A detergent and a surfactant. Order from a chemical supply house or from Continental Chemical Co.

SODIUM PERBORATE   A disinfectant when used in tooth preparations and a neutralizing agent when used in cold-wave preparations. Buy it at the drug store.

SORBO   A 70 percent solution of sorbitol (see *Arlacels*).

SPAN 60   Sorbitan monostearate (see *Arlacels*).

SPAN 80   Sorbitan monooleate (see *Arlacels*).

SPERMACETI   A soft, crystalline wax obtained from the head cavity of the sperm whale. Spermaceti imparts a firm consistency to fat mixtures. Because the sperm whale is considered to be an endangered species, a synthetic spermaceti is now available that has virtually identical physical properties. It is recommended for all formulas in this book calling for spermaceti wax. Buy it at the drug store or from a supplier of waxes, such as the Cornelius Wax Refining Corp.

STANNIC OXIDE   A high quality abrasive. Buy it from your druggist or order from a chemical supply house.

STARCHES, CORN, RICE, ETC   Used in cosmetics as thickeners as well as materials to absorb moisture. They are soothing to the skin and are frequently used in powders. Buy them in food or health food stores.

STEARIC ACID   A fatty acid occurring naturally in animal fats and tallow, as well as in many vegetable oils. It has always been used in making soaps and is the raw material from which many cooking oils come. Uncombined stearic acid, in cosmetic creams, provides the pearliness and firmness which are common in vanishing creams. In combination with an alkali (such as triethanolamine), it reacts to form a salt which is the basis for soaps. Buy it at the drug store.

STEARYL ALCOHOL   Acts as a skin emollient. It prevents degreasing of the outermost layer of the skin. Available at the drug store.

SUN SCREEN   A material which absorbs ultraviolet sun radiation, thus protecting the skin from rays which cause burning. An example is phenyl salicylate crystals (salol).

SURFACTANT   A substance that, when dissolved in a liquid, tends to concentrate on its surface and reduces the surface tension of the liquid. This property is valuable in the manufacture of emulsions.

TALC   Hydrated magnesium silicate which occurs naturally. Italian and French varieties are considered the best for cosmetic use. Talc has good "slip," permitting powders to spread easily, but has poor covering power, hence zinc or titanium oxide is usually incorporated with talc in face powders. Buy it at the drug store.

THYMOL   A crystalline substance which is a germicide, frequently used in mouth washes, deodorants, and hair lotions. Available at the drug store.

TITANIUM DIOXIDE   A white powder, which, when dispersed in creams, covers skin imperfections. It is also used in conjunction with colored pigments to modify colors. Your druggist may have it; if not, order from a chemical supply house or manufacturer of cosmetic colorants such as those listed under *Pigments*.

TRAGACANTH, GUM   A vegetable mucin which forms a stable mucilage with water. Its properties are similar to those of lecithin. Readily available at the drug store.

TRIETHANOLAMINE   A weak base often used with stearic acid to convert the acid to a salt (stearate), becoming a base for soap. It is characterized by low alkalinity and freedom from skin-irritating characteristics. Ask your druggist to order triethanolamine from his supplier if he doesn't carry it. You may also purchase it from a chemical supply house. (See also *Stearic acid*.)

TRIETHANOLAMINE LAURYL SULFATE   A good detergent having excellent wetting properties. Ask your druggist to order it for you from his supplier or from Continental Chemical Co. (Of course you may order direct if you prefer.)

TWEEN 20   Polyoxyethylene sorbitan monolaurate (see *Arlacels*).

TWEEN 60   Polyoxyethylene sorbitan monostearate (see *Arlacels*).

TWEEN 80   Polyoxyethylene sorbitan monooleate (see *Arlacels*).

VETIVERT   An essential oil used in the manufacture of cosmetics. An imitation product is available. Buy it from a supplier of perfume concentrates.

WETTING AGENT   Used in mixing solids with liquids (see *Surfactant*).

WHEAT-GERM OIL   Rich in vitamin E, vitamin A, vitamin D, and certain of the B vitamins, polyunsaturated fatty acids, lecithin, estrogenic substances, and other steroids. It is used in cosmetics because of its emollient qualities. In addition, it is sometimes used in cosmetics because of its vitamin and estrogenic content. Buy it at your food or health food store.

WITCH HAZEL (Hamamelis water) A mild astringent. The astringent effect of this and other vegetable extracts is due to the presence of tannic acid. It is frequently used as a cosmetic as it comes from the bottle, and is valued for its soothing, refreshing characteristics. Available at all drug and some food stores.

ZINC OXIDE Used in powders and creams because of its covering power. It also has astringent and sun screen applications. Buy it at the drugstore.

ZINC PEROXIDE Used in cosmetic formulations for its astringent characteristics. You may find it at the drugstore; if not, order it from a chemical supply house.

ZINC STEARATE A fine powder that increases the adhesive capabilities of face, baby, and body powders. Available at the drugstore or from a chemical supply house.

APPENDIX B

Suppliers

ATLAS CHEMICAL INDUSTRIES (Spans, Tweens, Arlacels, Sorbo, (G-1790 and G-2162)
Wilmington, Del. 19899
You may obtain literature from the above address, but small-lot quantities of the products named above should be ordered from EMULSION ENGINEERING, INC., *or* VAN WATERS AND ROGERS UNITED CO.

BAKER CASTOR OIL CO. (Sulfonated oils)
40 Avenue A
Bayonne, N.J. 07002

CALAVO GROWERS OF CALIFORNIA (avocado oil)
Box 3486 Terminal Annex
Los Angeles, Calif. 90058

COLE-PARMER (general laboratory supplies)
7425 North Oak Park Ave.
Chicago, Ill. 60648

CONTINENTAL CHEMICAL CO. (detergents, surfactants)
270 Clifton Blvd.
Clifton, N.J. 07015

CORNELIUS WAX REFINING CORP. (waxes)
1711 Elizabeth Ave. W.
Linden, N.J. 07036

CURTIN SCIENTIFIC CO. (general laboratory supplies)
P.O. Box 1546
Houston, Tex. 77001

EMULSION ENGINEERING, INC. (Spans, Tweens, Arlacels, Sorbo,
G-1790, and G-2162)
480 Bennett Rd.
Elk Grove Village, Ill. 60007

FISHER SCIENTIFIC CO. (general laboratory supplies)
717 Forbes Ave.
Pittsburgh, Pa. 15219

FLORASYNTH LABORATORIES, INC. (fragrances)
900 Van Nest Ave.
Bronx, N.Y. 10462

GAF CORP. (sulfonated oils)
140 W. 51st St.
New York, N.Y. 10020

LEEBEN COLOR AND CHEMICAL CO., INC. (cosmetic colorants)
103 Lafayette St.
New York, N.Y. 10013

NORDA ESSENTIAL OIL AND CHEMICAL CO. (fragrances)
475 Tenth Ave.
New York, N.Y. 10018

SUN CHEMICAL CORP. (cosmetic colorants)
Pigments Dept.
441 Tompkins Ave.
Rosebank
Staten Island, N.Y. 10305

SYNFLEUR SCIENTIFIC LABORATORIES, INC. (fragrances)
Monticello, N.Y. 12701

VAN DYK AND COMPANY, INC. (fragrances)
11 William St.
Belleville, N.J. 07109

VAN WATERS AND ROGERS (general laboratory supplies and chemicals)
P.O. Box 3200
San Francisco, Calif. 94119
(*Also, Ann Arbor, Mich.; Atlanta, Ga.; Baltimore, Md.; Bronx, N.Y.; Buffalo, N.Y.; Cambridge, Mass.; Columbus, Ohio; Albequerque, N.M.; Anchorage, Alaska; Denver, Colo.; El Paso, Tex.; Honolulu, Hawaii; Los Angeles, Calif.; Phoenix, Ariz.; Portland, Ore.; Salt Lake City, Utah; San Diego, Calif.; Seattle, Wash.; Tucson, Ariz.; West Sacramento, Calif.; Rochester, N.Y.*)

WELCH, HOLME AND CLARK CO., INC. (sulfonated oils)
1000 South 4th St.
Harrison, N.J. 07029

NOTE: In addition to the sources listed, there are chemical supply houses throughout the country. Check your telephone yellow pages for sources in your area.

Index

after-shave lotions, 129, 138
After-shave Stick, 136–137
animal fats
  cosmetics made with, 3
anointment, 5
anti-perspirants, 113, 122–123
  cream, 122
  liquid, 123
aromatic waters, 45
astringent lotion, 45, 59–60
Avocado Cream, 63–64
Avocado Moisturizer, 58
avocado oil, 27, 149

Baby Powder, 65
barley flour, 7
Bath Oil, 114, 124
bath preparations, 114, 123–
  126
  Bath Oil, 124
  Bath Salts, 124

Body Oil, 125–126
bubble powders, 114
  Foam Bath, 123
beautification, 76–106, 128
beeswax, 22, 149
Blush Rouge, 93–94
Body Oil, 125–126
borax, 22, 149
boric acid, 38, 149
butter, 7

chalk, 7
cleansing cosmetics, 12, 43,
  44, 52–55
Cleansing Cream No. 1, 52–
  53
Cleansing Cream No. 2, 53
Cleansing Lotion, 54–55
Cleansing Milk, 55
Cleopatra, 1, 6, 45

cold creams, 40–41, 48–51
  basic, 48–50
  theatrical, 51
cologne
  cream, 104–105
  men's, 143–144
colorants, 36–37, 113
cosmetic fashions, 2, 4, 7–8, 78, 129
cosmetic manufacture
  basic rules of, 21–22, 25–32
  cost of, xv, 12, 15–16, 59, 105–106
  equipment for, 25–28
  experimentation with, 18–19
  heating in, 29, 31–32
  laws governing, 20–24, 36
  pigments used in, 36–37, 87–101
  precautions taken in, 21–23, 29–31
cosmetic safety, 13, 18, 20–24
cosmetics
  animal fats used in, 3
  colorants, 36–37
  damage from, 13, 22
  delaying effects of age with, 69–71
  history of, 1–9, 40–41, 45, 79, 82, 113, 128
  labeling of, 23–24
  men's, 127–144
  moral issues of, 7–8, 79
  packaging of, 31–32, 105
  perfuming of, 33–36

  preservatives for, 37–39
  psychological effects of, 10, 11, 34–35, 41, 45, 108–109
  purity of, 23
  religious use of, 5, 6
cream cologne, 104–105
cream makeup, 89–90
creams, 29–30, 44–45, 48–59, 132
  All-Purpose, 51–52
  Avocado Moisturizer, 58
  Basic Cold, No. 1, 48–49
  Basic Cold, No. 2, 49–50
  Basic Cold, No. 3, 50
  cleansing, 43, 44, 52–55
  Cleansing, No. 1, 52–53
  Cleansing, No. 2, 53
  Cleansing Lotion, 54–55
  Cleansing Milk, 55
  cold, 44, 48–51
  Dry-Skin Vanishing, 57–58
  face, 43
  Liquid Cleansing, 54
  Lubricating, 58–59
  massage, 141–142
  men's, 141–142
  men's hair, 133–134
  Mentholated Massage, 141–142
  "miracle," 24
  "nourishing," 24
  preservatives for, 38
  Protective Sun, 141
  Theatrical Cold, 51
  Simple Vanishing, 56–57

vanishing, 43, 44, 56–58
cream shampoo, 115

deodorants, 109, 122–123, 129, 132, 142–143
    Deodorant Foot Powder, 143,
    Deodorant Stick, 142
    men's, 142–143
deodorants and anti-perspirants
    Anti-perspirant Cream, 122
    Liquid Anti-perspirant, 123
depilatory, 7
dyes, 22, 113

Electric Pre-shave Lotion, 136
Elizabeth I, 7
emollients, 48–51, 151
emulsions, 15, 29–30, 40–41, 44, 151
enfleurage, 87, 104
equipment, 25–28
    sources of supply, 25–26, 162–164
eye makeup, 82–83, 96–101
    brow pencils and liners, 83
    Cake Mascara No. 1, 98–99
    Cake Mascara No. 2, 99–100
    Cream Eye Shadow, 96–97
    Eye Makeup Remover, 101
    mascara, 83, 98–101
    Mascara Crayon, 100–101
    Powder Eye Shadow, 97–98
    preservatives for, 38

Remover, 83, 101
eye shadow
    Cream, 82–83, 96–97
    Powder, 82–83, 97–98

face creams, 43, 48–58, 87
face makeup, 80–82, 87–96
    Blush Rouge, 93–94
    Cream Makeup, 89–90
    Face Powders, 91–93
    foundation, 80, 87–88
    Foundation Cream, 87–88
    Lipstick, 94–96
    Liquid Makeup, 90–91
    Pigmented Foundation Cream, 88
    powders, 80–81, 91–93
    rouge, 81
Face Powders, 91–93
Federal Food, Drug, and Cosmetic Act (1938), 23
Foam Bath, 114, 123–124
foot powder, deodorant, 143
foundation cream, 87–88
    pigmented, 88
foundation makeups, 42, 80, 87–88
fragrances, 3, 85–87, 127, 129
    ambergris, 3, 148
    civet, 3, 150
    Cream Cologne, 104–105
    henna flowers, 3
    homemade perfumes, 104
    honey, 3
    iris root, 3
    men's, 127, 129

fragrances (*cont'd.*)
  musk, 3, 155
  "Pure Joy," 105–106
  wine, 3
fucus (rouge), 7

gelatin mask, 61–62
Glycerin and Rose Water, 17,
  30, 41, 63
grooming, 5, 41, 107–126, 128

hair care, 22, 108–110, 133–
  134
hair conditioners, 111, 119
hair preparations, 11, 111,
  129, 133–134
  Clear Hairdressing, 134
  Cream Shampoo, 115–116
  Hair Cream, 133–134
  Hair-Set Preparation, 119–
    120
  Hot Oil Conditioner, 119
  Liquid Shampoo, 114–115
  (Simple) Oil Shampoo, 116
  Soap Shampoo, 117–119
hand creams and lotions, 62–
  64
  Avocado Cream, 63–64
  Deluxe Hand Cream, 64
  Glycerin and Rose Water,
    63
  Simple Hand Cream (Oily),
    62
hand preparations, 131, 138–
  140

Extra-rich Lubricant, 138–
  139
Hand Cleaner No. 1, 139–
  140
Hand Cleaner No. 2, 140
health care, 10, 13, 20–21, 22,
  42, 107–108
heating, 29, 31–32
henna, 6, 33
Hentawi, 10, 11
horomones, 69–75

ingredients
  list of, 147–171
  buying, 21, 26–27, 36, 38
  measuring, 27–28, 35–36
  mixing, 29–31
  sources of supply, 26–27,
    162–164
  substitutions, 22
  "technical" grade, 21
iodine, white tincture of, 38

Johnson, Lynda Bird, 78

kaolin, 153
Kaolin Mask, 60–61
kohl, 1

labeling of cosmetics, 23–24
lanolin, 3, 11, 153
lipstick, 11, 79, 81–82, 94–
  96
Liquid Makeup, 90
Liquid Shampoo, 114–115
litmus paper, 39, 154

Loren, Sophia, 78
lotions
  astringent, 45
  cleansing, 54–55
  skin, 59–60
lubricating creams, 11, 15, 42, 44, 58–59, 129

mascara, 83, 98–101
  Cake, No. 1, 98–99
  Cake, No. 2, 99–100
  Crayon, 100–101
masks, 42, 45, 60–62
  Gelatin Mask, 61–62
  Kaolin Mask, 60–61
massage cream, 141–142
Masters, George, 78
measurement of ingredients, 27–28
men's cosmetics, 127–144
  clear hairdressing, 130–131
  cologne, 143–144
  deodorants, 142–143
  hair cream, 130, 133–134
  mentholated massage cream, 141–142
methyl paraben, 38, 154
milk, 7, 55
  Cleansing, 55
mineral oil, 22
"miracle" creams, 24
mixing, 29–31
Moisturizer, Avocado, 58
mouth preparations, 112–113, 120–122
  Mouthwash, 121–122

Toothpaste, 120
Tooth Powder, 120–121
Mouthwash, 112–113, 121–122

Nail-Buffing Paste, 11, 18, 102–103
Nail Polish Remover, 85, 103
nail preparations, 83–85, 102–103
  lacquers, 84
  Nail Buffing Paste, 102–103
  Nail Polish Remover, 103
NF (National Formulary), 21
"nourishing" creams, 24

oils, 2, 3
  aromatic, 4
  avocado, 27, 149
  ben, 3
  castor, 3, 150
  colocynth, 3
  lemon, 35
  lime, 35
  "magic," 6
  olive, 3, 41, 155
  orange, 35
  perfume, 35, 156
  radish, 3
  religious, 5, 6
  rose, 157
  sesame, 3, 27, 157
  wheat-germ, 27, 160
Oil Shampoo, Simple, 116–117
ointments, 2, 4

packaging cosmetics, 32
packs, *see* masks
pastes, 11, 18, 30–31, 102–103
perfumes, 3, 4, 33–36, 85–87,
    129, 143–144
  artificial flower oils, 86
  finished, 86–87
  homemade, 104
  isolates, 86
  men's, 132–133, 143–144
  natural, 86
  synthetic, 86
perfumes and flavorings, 3,
    33, 35, 152, 156, 157
Pigmented Foundation Cream,
    88
pigments, 36–37, 80–101, 156
Pignatelli, Princess Luciana, 9
pollution, 45
powders, 30–31, 65–66
  baby, 65
  face, 80–81, 91–93
  foot, 143
  talcum, 65–66
preservatives, 37–39
protective cosmetics, 11, 43,
    87–88, 141
pumice, 7
"Pure Joy," 105–106

red ocher, 6, 33
rouge, 7, 79, 81, 93–94

salicylic acid, 38
shampoos, 111, 114–119
  cream, 115–116

liquid, 114–115
oil, 116
soap, 117–119
shaving preparations, 129,
    130–131, 134–138
  After-shave Lotion, 138
  After-shave Stick, 136
  Brushless Shaving Cream
    No. 1, 134–135
  Brushless Shaving Cream
    No. 2, 135–136
  Electric Pre-shave Lotion,
    136
skin care, 20–21, 40–68, 70–
    75
skin cleansing, 41–42
skin freshener, 60
skin lotions
  Astringent Lotion, 59–60
  Skin Freshener, 60
skin lubrication, 41–43
Soap Shampoo, 117–119
sources of supply
  equipment, 25–26, 162–164
  ingredients, 21, 26–27, 162–
    164
Sun Cream Protective, 141
Sun Tan Oil, 67
sun tan preparations, 43, 47–
    48, 67–68
suppliers, xv, 27
  list of, 162–164

Talcum Powders, 65–66
tanning preparations, 67–68
  Sun Tan Cream, 67–68

Sun Tan Oil, 67
thermometer, 31–32
Toothpaste, 109, 112, 120
Tooth Powder, 112, 120–121
Tutankhamen, King, 4

unguents, 2, 4
    religious, 5
USP (United States Pharma-
        copeia), 21

vanishing creams, 11, 42, 56–
        58
    dry-skin, 57–58
    simple, 56–57
vitamins, 63, 69–75

waxes, 28
white lead, 7
wine, 3, 7

zinc oxide, 129, 161